How Thousands of My Arthritis Patients Regained Their Health

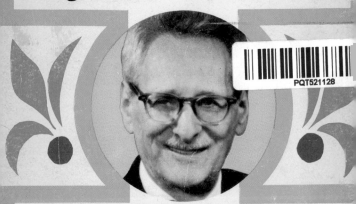

MAX WARMBRAND, N.D., D.C., D.O.

An internationally-known naturopathic
physician's drugless program for restoring
arthritis and rheumatism sufferers
to vital new health through
planned exercise and a diet of natural foods

ARC

$1.65

165

How Thousands of My Arthritis Patients Regained Their Health

MAX WARMBRAND, N.D., D.C., D.O.

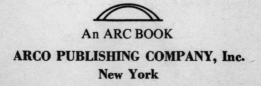

An ARC BOOK
ARCO PUBLISHING COMPANY, Inc.
New York

First ARC Printing, 1971

An ARC Book
Published by Arco Publishing Company, Inc.
219 Park Avenue South, New York, N. Y. 10003
by arrangement with Parker Publishing Co. Inc.

ISBN 0-668-02488-7

Printed in the United States of America

FOREWORD BY A DOCTOR
OF MEDICINE

In explaining how the utilization of nature's healing and re-building laws has helped thousands of his arthritis patients regain their health, Dr. Warmbrand renders much needed service to the millions who are suffering from this extremely painful and crippling disease and who have been seeking in vain the help which they need. In this book, Dr. Warmbrand portrays the central theme of adherence to nature, the reward for which is health and a greater enjoyment of living. His is the system of total rehabilitation which he has practiced all his professional life—a system which embraces healthful nutrition, the proper use of our knowledge of physical education and certainly not least, recognition of the power of the mind in reassuring the sick and inspiring confidence toward the goal of getting well. This end result becomes so much more facilitated when a state of confidence, tranquility, and peace of mind has been given to the ill by the sincere, untiring efforts of a sympathetic physician. This method thus employs the concept of treating the individual as a whole—a living synthesis of body, mind, and spirit, and represents the direct antithesis of fragmentation or the treatment of parts.

Dr. Warmbrand has penetrated the very heart and soul of nature and, having discovered her vital laws, makes an eloquent and powerful plea for all to follow the laws of the Mother of all living things. This benefits not only those already afflicted by arthritis but also protects against its onset by preventing ill health generally.

It is quite relevant at this point to make known to the reader that the author, a victim in his youth of a so-called incurable ailment, succeeded by the methods described in this book, to bring himself back to a state of vigorous health, and while doing this gained the insight which enabled him to provide this valuable help to many thousands of arthritis sufferers who came to him for help and guidance.

In this book Dr. Warmbrand has given all of himself—in these pages is the true reflection of this man. It is the creation of a sincere and honorable doctor whose greatest desire is to heal the sick. In his fifty years as a physician, working in cooperation with the healing laws of nature, he has brought new life to many, in some instances bordering even on the miraculous.

This book is revealing of all this. Anyone suffering from the painful and agonizing disease called arthritis will be stimulated and inspired with new hope and a healthful attitude toward life.

Joseph L. Kaplowe, M.D.

HOW THIS BOOK CAN HELP YOU

The many victims of arthritis who keep suffering from the encroaching effects of this extremely painful and crippling disease are always searching for a plan, a program, or a remedy that can get them well or at least make their life more bearable. If you are one of the many millions who are suffering from this disease and really wish to get well, this book can be the answer for you. It is based upon my more than fifty years of experience as a naturopathic, osteopathic and chiropractic physician treating all types of arthritis, from the very simplest to those which are already accompanied by untold agony and crippling. It explains how the disease originates, it clarifies many of the points that you have to know if you are to succeed in overcoming this body-wracking illness. It outlines in full detail the care that has helped countless thousands of sufferers from this disease of arthritis to renewed health and usefulness and that can do the same for you.

My methods are completely drugless. The programs presented in this book call for a completely non-drug approach. At no time are there any costly remedies required. The basic principle is to became allied with Nature and apply natural methods to help you.

How this book can save you money. Practically everything suggested in this book may be performed right in your own home. No expensive medicines, no high hospitalization costs, no frightening doctor bills. Where possible, the advice and guidance of a physician specializing in natural healing is recommended, but the program outlined calls for no outlay in expensive drugs, no costly trips to spas or health resorts, nor frequent and costly visits to the doctor's office. And what is most valuable, results in most cases are not only positive and constructive,—they can often be actually phenomenal!

The plan is easy to follow. This book explains in clear, easily understandable terms how you can go about rebuilding your health and rid yourself of this crippling and highly debilitating disease. There are no "instant cures," no "crash programs." But, and this is the point that is most essential, what you must do for yourself if you really wish to get well is revealed in clear, simple language. The book presents a step-by-step program towards total and complete health restoration, and when you follow this program in a consistent and faithful way, satisfying results are inevitable.

Side effects from drugs avoided. Because these methods are drugless, you avoid many needless complications or drug-induced side effects. The almost miraculous benefits are derived because the whole program is based not on artificial aids and remedies, but on an all-natural program of health building. Your body is slowly cleansed of its toxic elements and then gradually restored to healthy functioning, and this ultimately leads to total rehabilitation of your health.

The method is surprisingly simple. All it takes is just a day-to-day program that you can easily adopt and follow. The rewards in most instances are so striking that they are almost unbelievable. No special complicated apparatus, no costly equipment is required. Whatever you need is easily obtainable at the neighborhood stores. All you have to do is adopt this plan and follow it consistently and faithfully.

You enjoy complete privacy. Nearly everything you have to do as called for in this book can be performed right in the privacy of your own home. No one need know what you are trying to do. You may actually wish to do it without discussing it with others to avoid being led astray or being thrown off the right path. You are shown how to organize the healing forces that exist *within your own body* by making simple adjustments in your day-to-day living habits, and you are inspired to be determined to make total rebuilding your goal.

Nature cures when drugs fail. The many case histories presented in this book show how nature can still help you even when everything else that you have heretofore tried has failed to provide satisfactory help. The plans presented in this book, if followed consistently, enable the healing forces of your body to get at the causes of the disease and uproot them. While drugs temporarily suppress painful symptoms, they do not eradicate the basic causes of the disease, and the disease only continues to get worse. In this book you will be shown how you can make use of the dynamic healing forces always present within your own body to help you conquer your arthritis and gain a vibrant life of renewed health and well-being.

Max Warmbrand, N.D., D.C., D.O.

CONTENTS

10

1

EVIDENCE THAT
ARTHRITIS SUFFERERS
CAN GET WELL

This is a book for people of all ages, in all walks of life, who want to enjoy a life that is free from aches, pains, premature aging, and degeneration of mind and body. It is written to help those who are victims of the many different forms of arthritis and rheumatism.

I say there are many different forms of arthritis and rheumatism because in my half century of practice as an osteopathic, naturopathic, and chiropractic physician I have treated thousands who have complained of muscular stiffness, aching pains, sore shoulders, tennis elbows, swollen and painful wrists and hands, bursitis, and spasms, and found that arthritis has many outward signs of its presence.

It has become clear that in most cases, arthritis and rheumatism are not single, definable diseases, but names loosely applied to many disorders in and around the joints.

Whether you suffer from a sore back when you bend over, or whether you are confined to a wheelchair, this book can help you. It is different from other books because the method of healing that I have found so successful for many thousands of cases in my lifelong professional practice, is based not upon the use of drugs but upon the use of measures that work with the healing powers of the body.

THE FALLACY OF DRUGS FOR ARTHRITIS

All drugs, whether they are simple aspirin or cortisone, only mask the disease. *They do not get rid of it.* An arthritis sufferer who takes drugs still has his arthritis (which often grows increasingly worse as the years go on), even though the mechanism that transmits the sensation of pain is temporarily blocked out and the patient lives under the illusion that he has been helped.

A warm, dry climate may be helpful, but the arthritis still remains although the pain may temporarily become more bearable. In my professional practice I have treated thousands of arthritis patients who at one time or another thought that by running away from home or by changing to a warmer climate they would get better, only to find out later that their condition grew steadily worse. A balmy-weather location does help you relax, but the arthritis still remains. I have helped many thousands of arthritis sufferers by putting them on a drug-free plan, by prescribing special exercises, a dietary regimen that includes natural, wholesome body- and health-building foods, a regulated plan to help drain and eliminate internal toxic waste products, friction baths, home applicable manipulative measures, various water applications, a unique mono-diet program, and other highly successful self-help measures.

Many arthritis sufferers who had been slaves to drugs while their disease kept growing constantly worse, were freed from their painful symptoms and became completely well when they adopted and consistently followed the program that I outlined for them.

HOW ANDREW W. RECOVERED FROM ARTHRITIS AFTER THREE YEARS OF HOPELESS SUFFERING

When you read the dramatic case history of Andrew, you will see why I am so enthusiastic about natural methods of care. Andrew is an electronic engineer. He had been suffering from arthritis for some years, and for the last three years his condition had been getting considerably worse. His illness started originally with just a slight ache in his back, then his joints became a little stiff. He had a slight swelling of his fingers. Little by little the symptoms became worse. For the last three years he was barely able to walk and had to give up his work.

He had tried everything in the way of medicines and injections. He was given cortisone, he received gold injections, and he lived on a wide variety of different aspirins and other pain killers. He would get some temporary relief at times, but the pains and suffering continued to grow worse.

Andrew said that he could not raise his arms. "I could not put any pressure on the screw driver or pliers or any of the other tools I used at my work, and every time I sat down and had to get up it hurt so much that I felt like fainting. And the money I spent trying to get well! It did me no good. I was only continuing to get worse with each day."

He said that his neck became so stiff and painful, it felt as if it were nailed down solidly. He could barely move his head and neck. His hips, his elbows, his neck, his feet, and his shoulders too, were agonizingly painful, every move was sheer torture.

Abstain from All Drugs

This is my first rule. Then, I put him on a special diet plan which called for the elimination of all artificial foods (such as those made from white flour, white sugar, sharp irritating spices and seasonings or those containing artificial colorings or flavors), and also all stimulating beverages including coffee, tea, cola drinks, liquor, and the like.

Developing Good Eating Habits. He was told to eat slowly, to chew his food thoroughly so that all vital nutrients would be extracted. He was told to eat only when hungry and not to over-eat.

Internal Cleansing Plan. Toxic waste substances, internal sludge and mucus, set up chain reactions that lead to arthritic symptoms. Toxic or health damaging substances accumulating in the body often lead to the development of this affliction. Therefore, I placed Andrew on an internal cleansing plan that included the consumption of fresh raw fruit and vegetable drinks, and the use of toxin-eliminative health measures. Laxatives became unnecessary. With good food, good eating habits, and retraining, constipation was eliminated. Established regularity meant that internal wastes were being removed and the internal organs and parts of his body were restored to a more normal condition.

Freedom from Tension. Since nervous tension often leads to arthritis, I suggested that Andrew get rid of his artificial tranquilizers and overcome his tensions the natural, easy way. He was to dissolve two glasses of epsom salt in a tub of hot water and bathe in it every night before retiring. He was instructed to keep the hot water dripping in while he was in the tub to make sure that the temperature of the bath was maintained at an even rate, and comfortably and pleasantly hot.

A Good Night's Sleep. Following the bath, Andrew was to retire immediately and go to sleep. The hot epsom salt baths encourage elimination by way of the skin and the kidneys, promote better circulation, help relieve nervous tension, and loosen up tense and tightened muscles. The baths encourage better body functioning. Patients often perspire after the bath, and this is only desirable and helpful.

Deep Breathing Exercises. All methods of healing throughout the ages have recognized the beneficial effects of deep breathing. I then recommended that Andrew follow a specific deep breathing exercise program. Deep breathing exercises increase the intake of oxygen into the body and promote the elimination of toxins by way of the lungs, while these and various other physical exercises adhered to daily, promote better circulation and help in general body rejuvenation. In arthritis, the need to break up internal congestion and stagnation is great. The deep breathing and other regulated physical exercises that I prescribed for him are very valuable for those who suffer from arthritis or related disorders.

An Abundance of Rest and Sleep. I also insisted that he obtain an abundance of rest and sleep. He needed to develop poise and emotional control as part of a better and more regulated way of living. Rest, sleep, the development of poise and emotional control help to rebuild the health of the body and establish better overall body functioning.

Elimination of Harmful Habits. I also pointed out to him that since health-debilitating habits interfere with recovery and cause only more pain and suffering, they had to be given up. Smoking, drinking, late hours, overexposure, lack of sufficient sleep and rest, the use of artificial sweets and bleached flour products, all have a detrimental effect on health and aggravate arthritis. And, as I said before, Andrew gave up aspirin, cortisone, all other pain-dulling medicines. There was no magic in these drugs, and while they provide a certain amount of temporary relief, they only mask the disease and lead to a more severe form of arthritis.

Furthermore, nobody can predict what the long-term effects of these drugs are likely to be; any remedy that artificially suppresses pain, in the long run also undermines the health-restorative powers of the body.

During the three months that Andrew came to see me, I also applied certain specific manipulative treatments. These helped to loosen up tightened muscles, promoted better circulation to the stiff, rigid and congested joints, and helped to relax his body. In a later chapter, I refer to these manipulative techniques and explain how arthritis sufferers can use many of them with great benefit right in the privacy of their own home.

At first Andrew was skeptical, but since he was so badly crippled with the disease he decided he had nothing to lose (except his arthritis) and everything to gain. So, he cooperated with me in my method of helping Nature overcome his disease.

ANDREW COULD HARDLY WALK

When Andrew began with this care, he could barely walk! Every step was torture. His pains when getting out of bed were indescribable, and they continued to get progressively worse. He could drive his car, but to get in and out of it, was sheer misery. He was almost bedridden. So I started by explaining to him that if he wanted to get rid of this crippling disease, he would have to follow the program that I would outline for him. I had used this program most successfully in many thousands of cases, and he too could be helped just like those thousands of others who overcame their illness and returned to a normal and pain-free life.

He agreed to cooperate and the plan decribed above was prepared for him. As weeks went on, he regained increasing use of his limbs and freedom from pain. By the time the three-month program was ended, he was back at work. He could walk, bend, twist, and turn—and no pain! His hands, his arms, and his shoulders could move freely—something that is very important to his work. All movements were without pain.

Nature Must Have Time to Heal

At this point let me make one point clear. While Andrew, just as thousands of other arthritis sufferers who adopted the program that I am outlining in this book, showed a remarkable degree of improvement in such a short period of time, none who suffer from this disease must delude themselves into thinking that although they are feeling better, their disease has already been completely overcome.

Arthritis is a disease that usually takes years to develop, and three months of even the best of care cannot uproot it in its entirety. Those who suffer from the simpler forms of the disease may regain a high level of good health after following this approach for only a few months, possibly six or eight months. Those, however, in whom the disease had already become deeply rooted, may require intensive care over a much longer period of time, sometimes even two years or longer before they obtain all the help they need. This is a point that sufferers from arthritis must always keep in mind so that they persist with the needed care even after they have already regained a considerable amount of health.

THE CRIPPLED PATIENT WHO MADE A SLOW BUT STEADY RECOVERY

In Claire C.'s case it took a great deal longer before her body-wracking and crippling arthritis was uprooted, but what made her especially happy were the many added benefits that she derived from this care while her ailment was being eradicated.

Claire C. was 57 when she came to see me. She had been suffering from arthritis for many years. Her whole body was badly crippled. Her back, her knees, her hands, her shoulders, were badly deformed and extremely painful. She had been under the care of many doctors and was treated with many medicines.

Drugs Did Little Good. Among the drugs that she was kept on were indocin, cortisone, gold injections, a variety of other drugs. None was of any real help. She continued to grow consistently worse. She became badly crippled and was in deep misery.

Case History Shows Side Effects. It was difficult to determine when and how her arthritis actually started, but as it increased, so did her other ailments. Her pains were most agonizing and she also suffered from poor circulation in the feet for years. Her knees, her hands, her shoulders, her back, were badly deformed from the disease. Her badly swollen knees had to be tapped regularly to remove the fluid that accumulated in them. Tapping provided temporary relief, but Claire C. had to go back to the doctor to have this repeated regularly about three times a year.

Drugs Mask Disease but Condition Worsens. She also continued to take her drugs, and then one day, upon examination it was discovered that she was suffering from glaucoma, a dangerous eye disorder in which the fluid pressure within the eyeball is markedly increased. The doctor immediately discontinued the use of aralen, one of the drugs that she was kept on at this time and that is known to have a damaging effect on the eyes. With the discontinuance of aralen, the pains reawakened in even more severe form. The pains in her legs, shoulders and wrists showed up all over again in the most intense way.

A Series of Controlled Gold Injections Were Started

But arthritis pains and side effects still continued. After four series of gold injections and indocin, Claire C. now began to complain of stomach disorders. When gold and indocin were discontinued, her stomach problems cleared up.

The doctor told her that she would have to take drugs for relief of pain for the rest of her life since arthritis is incurable, but that drugs will help her to live with it. Nothing was said about adopting the necessary measures to help her get rid of the disease.

My Treatment Begins. Claire came to see me as a last resort and I have often thought how much misery she could have avoided had she come to me during the early stages of her illness. Immediately I put her on a program of controlled fasting, corrective exercises, the hot epsom salt baths, natural foods, a complete hygienic living program. It took close to two years until most of her pains and aches disappeared.

Added Benefits

Her Nails Began to Grow Back. One day, just a few months after following my program, Claire discovered that her fingernails were growing in again. Previously her nails would split, peel, but they never seemed to grow. Now they are strong and healthy again, and keep growing regularly.

Her Eyelashes Grew in Again. The illness caused her eyelashes to fall out. Under my care, they started to grow in again. They became so beautiful, many commented on the change.

Her Hair Became Lustrous and Shiny. Her hair became lustrous and shiny again. The natural care revitalized the entire body to the point where exteriorly too she began to show many healthful benefits, a reflection of the benefits that she derived as the health of the entire body was being rebuilt.

Improvement in Her Glaucoma Condition. Her serious eye condition began to show marked improvement. Her husband, an optometrist, had his wife's eyes checked regularly by an ophthalmologist who noticed that the pressure in her eyes showed a marked decrease.

Overall Rejuvenation. Claire became much younger in looks, much more vital. She started to walk straight and upright, something she couldn't do when she first came to see me. And all her other disorders began to clear up as her arthritis began to get better. One day I told her how much better she looked, how much straighter and taller she was, and she replied, "It was all those darn vegetables that you made me eat, that did it." And before she started with me, she never ate a vegetable, she hated them!

MY OWN PERSONAL EXPERIENCE

At a very young age, I began to suffer from t.b. (tuberculosis) of the joints and bones. I speak from my own personal as well as from professional experience when I say that sufferers from arthritis can get well. This type of joint disease (tuberculosis) is much more difficult than the type of joint disease known as arthritis, and no drugs or medicines could offer me any help. My choice was to resign myself to a state of hopelessness, invalidism and an early grave, or find a way that would provide the help I needed.

And so, I started the study of various healing sciences, and because of my own joint problem, I was particularly interested in finding out what could be done for those who suffered from the various diseases of the joints. I ultimately qualified in the various branches of natural healing, naturopathy, osteopathy, and chiropractic, and because of my own serious health problem I became my own first patient. This is how I helped myself and then helped others who suffered from the more common joint ailments such as arthritis and its related ills. All I had to do was to adopt this new approach to better health and to follow it consistently. Although it took a great deal of time before I succeeded in regaining my health, I ultimately conquered my own debilitating joint disease and thus became a living example of what natural healing can often accomplish even in seemingly hopeless afflictions.

Lung Scars

X-rays of my lungs disclosed the presence of scars, which indicates that during my childhood years I also suffered from tuberculosis of the lungs.

Worsening Condition. Acute fever attacks, agonizing pains, and severe crippling made me a complete invalid for long periods of time. My future looked grim and uncertain. Doctors knew that

I couldn't live long, and while living I would be practically an invalid.

That was when I started to look for an answer to my own health problem. Since I was young, I did not fully realize how seriously ill I was, and I was determined to get well. This is how I came upon the method of healing that I have applied most successfully in my own case and then with such phenomenal success in countless thousands of arthritis cases.

Because of the severity of my disease it took me a long time to regain my health, much longer than it ordinarily takes in arthritis. Altogether, it took about five years before I succeeded in conquering my illness completely. About three of those five years, I spent mostly on my back.

A stiff left hip and the scars on both of my legs in the places where abscesses formed and drained for years, are the only reminders of how desperately ill I was during those early years of my life and how near I was to death.

HOPE FOR ARTHRITIS SUFFERERS

Natural healing when correctly employed and persistently followed offers the only solutions to arthritis sufferers. Why? Because it discards the use of all pain and other symptom-suppressing drugs, and establishes a pattern of care that eliminates all the influences that give rise to the disease. It helps to correct all the weaknesses and disturbances that are part and parcel of the whole arthritis picture. While natural healing offers no specific remedy for arthritis, it nevertheless provides the care that rebuilds the overall health of the body and thereby uproots the arthritis condition. In other words, natural healing helps in rebuilding the health of the arthritis sufferer because it does not limit itself to the treatment of the disease itself, but rebuilds the health of the whole person. As the overall health of the patient is rebuilt, all the disorders associated with the disease as well as the arthritis itself, are overcome.

I feel that the experience I have gained in a professional healing practice extending over a period of more than fifty years, if faithfully and consistently applied, can do wonders for sufferers from arthritis. Countless thousands of arthritis sufferers, my patients, who have used this regimen, are living examples of how helpful natural healing can be in this greatly disabling disease, and if you apply this method in your own case, you too can obtain similar benefits.

This book contains the distillation of more than fifty years of practical experience in working towards the correction of this difficult ailment. My work started with my own illness, and then, after rebuilding my own health, helping others to regain theirs became a lifelong dedication.

Summary of the First Chapter: Points to Remember

1. Natural, wholesome foods, various kinds of water treatments, consistent home exercises, and other helpful natural care eliminate toxic wastes that accumulate in the system and that give rise to various arthritic disorders.
2. Freedom from tension, recuperative rest and sleep, and deep breathing, are vital in helping arthritis sufferers get well.
3. The methods in this book are drugless.

2

HOW ARTHRITIS
IS USUALLY THE OUTGROWTH OF
BASIC ILL HEALTH

The many different forms of arthritis and related rheumatic diseases can often be traced to malfunctioning of many of our internal organs. Internal toxemia in which the organs such as the liver, the kidneys, the pancreas, the intestines, the skin, as well as the endocrine systems, become clogged with acid-ash waste residues, usually initiates the disease known as arthritis. The preliminary disturbances that ultimately lead to the development of this crippling disorder often begin far away from the joints in the malfunctioning of the vital organs of the body.

Why Arthritis is Merely a Link in a Chain of Ill Health

Actually, arthritis (except when it develops as a result of trauma or accident) is merely one link in a chain of disorders that usually afflict sufferers from this disease. Arthritis is one link in a chain of ill health, and the various other disorders that often exist in association with it or that preceded its development are usually closely interrelated. Accumulations of internal wastes, faulty filtering of the kidneys, poor or inadequate liver functioning, failure of the skin to throw off toxic wastes, and other breakdowns of essential body processes, all add up to the retention of toxic end-products and the accumulation of acid waste substances. This leads to internal irritation and ultimately causes a derange-

29

ment in normal joint functioning with consequent destruction of the joint tissues.

ADVANCE WARNING SYMPTOMS

Irritants and toxins accumulating in the various organs and tissues of the body before the acute arthritis pains begin to appear, create many advance warning symptoms such as digestive disorders, poor circulation, constipation, poor liver and kidney functioning, and the like. Headaches, irritability, sleeplessness, and many other disorders often precede or accompany the onset of the disease. When the glandular-endocrine system is unable to function normally, it deprives the blood and skeletal system of vital oxygen and nourishment, and this brings about changes that favor the development of arthritis. It is well known among endocrinologists that the endocrine system regulates all bodily functioning—and this applies to all the internal organs as well as to the joints. When the glands are improperly nourished or their functions become deranged, body functioning becomes impaired and arthritis is one of the consequences.

REBUILDING FROM THE INSIDE

To defeat arthritis, the sufferer from this disease must embark upon a plan of rebuilding from within. He must look for more than just a remedy that relieves pains; he must adopt a plan of living and care that rebuilds the functioning of the glands as well as the health of the entire body.

How Gail Improved Her Health and Conquered Her Arthritis

When Gail first came to see me, she was about 20 years old. Many young people develop arthritis just like oldsters although they are not always aware of it, since the early stages of the disease are not always recognized. This is why I plead that the preliminary symptoms of ill health be heeded and that everything be done as soon as possible to check ill health in any form before it leads to more serious disorders.

Gail gave a history of previous attacks of bronchial asthma and frequently recurring choking of the throat, the condition doctors call *"globus hystericus,"* a nervous disorder that often accompanies certain digestive or nervous disorders. She was rather chubby, also extremely restless and irritable. At the least provocation and often even without provocation, Gail would become extremely unreasonable and upset and frequently go into tantrums.

When I examined Gail, I noted that her joints upon movement were making crunchy, creaking noises. They sounded like a discordant music box. Her knees seemed to be popping whenever I moved them. Many of her other joints, those of her shoulders and neck, also gave off creaking, cracking sounds.

Here already were clear signs of what was in store for Gail if she failed to overcome the various internal body disorders and rebuild the health of her whole body. Gail and her mother never paid any attention to these early joint symptoms simply because the disorder in the joints had not yet reached the point where it caused any difficulties. They were however concerned about her overall ill health and were especially worried about the consistent choking in her throat. And since there were no specific remedies that I could offer that could overcome Gail's specific internal disorders, I made it clear to them that if she was to get well she would have to adopt a complete health-restoration program and follow it faithfully. I also explained to them that the creaking and the grating of the joints indicated that the skeletal system had not been receiving an adequate supply of blood with its needed nutrients and oxygen, and that because of this failed to secrete the lubrication that was needed to keep the joints pliable and healthy. I further pointed out that this in time could lead to serious joint damage if she did not restore the functioning and health of her entire body.

Gail was also constipated, subject to frequent headaches, and was of a highly emotional and temperamental nature. She was addicted to sweets and rich desserts and never thought that the food she ate had much to do with her health. She did not exercise regularly, at certain times she would try to do too much, while at other times she would lock herself in her room and hardly do anything; and this too was an indication of her highly emotional state. She suffered from cold hands and feet. This was part of the malfunctioning of the hormonal system, and illustrated what effect it had on her circulation. That her blood sugar level was in constant fluctuation was evident. My program for Gail included the following health-restorative procedures:

1. *Keep warm.* The limbs and extremities should be kept warm and exposure to cold and dampness should be avoided. Create a feeling of warm pleasure.

2. *Rest.* An overactive body accumulates internal toxins that act as irritants to the joints and to all other parts of the body. Get as much rest as possible. One rule was that Gail was to rest following any activity that left her fatigued.

3. *Freedom from worry.* Emotional upsets and tensions aggravate the internal organs and hamper smooth functioning. Worries were to be avoided. Responsibilities were to be reduced.

4. *Improve diet.* Sugar and irritating spices create an acid-ash residue that leads to internal irritation. She was to avoid sweets, starches, "fluff" or artificial foods. Chemically treated preserved meats such as bacon, ham, corned beef, hot dogs, were not to be used. A moderate amount of fresh meat, broiled or baked (not fried!) was permissible. All excess fat was to be trimmed off to reduce the load on the digestive organs and to prevent the creation of too much toxic waste. Irritating sauces and condiments were not permitted. Salted and sharply seasoned foods had to be avoided. Vegetable flavoring such as sold in special diet shops, composed of wholesome ingredients, could be used.

5. *Avoid tobacco and alcohol.* Gail was not to smoke and was not to touch any liquor or any of the cola drinks. Tobacco contains harmful tars and causes a great deal of damage to the body. Liquor forces the liver and kidneys to work overtime to throw off the alcohol. It also "burns" these organs and impairs their functioning.

6. *Warmth was essential.* Keeping the body comfortably warm was another essential. During chilly weather, a flannel night gown and a flannel blanket were recommended.

7. *Restore bowel regularity*. Natural bowel movements are a "must" in the plan. For stubborn cases—and Gail was one—a glass of freshly squeezed apple juice taken upon an empty stomach in the morning was most helpful. Raw fruits, raw vegetables, and small amounts of whole grain foods, provide natural bulk. The body *must* dispose of its waste products, so regularity was most essential.

8. *Restore oxygen flow to head*. Quite often, headaches in such cases are traced to a choked off supply of oxygen needed to feed the brain. Headaches in Gail's case, were so prolonged that they caused a painful ache in the nape of her neck; in these joints, arthritis pockets were already beginning to set in. A few simple exercises were suggested. She was told to roll her head in a circle, right to left, then left to right, ten times. She was to do these exercises slowly, and stretch as far as she could. This helped to loosen up internal tension and also sent a flow of nutrient-carrying oxygen to the starved brain tissues. For rigidity and tautness between the shoulder blades or in the back of her head, this exercise was prescribed: Pull the shoulders up to the ears hard. Then while still holding them up, roll them forward with all your might and then thrust them back. Hold for ten seconds. Relax. Repeat ten times.

9. *Natural foods*. Gail's diet was to consist of natural foods prepared in as natural a manner as possible, also raw fruit and vegetable drinks because they provide good nutrition and help to flush out body impurities. One day a week she was to devote exclusively to either an all-day fruit juice diet or a vegetable juice one. Raw fruits or vegetables are very beneficial but for those arthritis sufferers who like a little more variety, stewed fruits or steamed vegetables for one of the meals is permissible. More success in building health, however, is derived from the raw, uncooked foods.

For a period of three months, Gail followed the preceding nine steps in rebuilding her internal health, and in doing this obtained a great deal of help.

But being young, and impulsive, she would occasionally indulge in sweets, soda pop, and processed meats such as hot dogs, hamburgers, and salami sandwiches. Whenever she "cheated," she fell victim to recurring head pains, body pains and ill health, and the choking would show up again. Furthermore, whenever she slipped back into faulty health habits the creaking in her joints recurred with greater intensity.

Gail Eight Years Later. This was about seven or eight years ago. After many beginnings, Gail finally realized that if she wanted to get well she would have to stop cheating. Today Gail is a vibrant, healthy young woman. The creaking or cracking of her joints is practically all gone. The choking in her throat is a thing of the past. She finally realized that if she was going to get well she would have to work with Nature. Nature does the healing when we provide the body with the help it needs. You cannot compromise with nature and get away with it. To get well, we must form a partnership with nature and not fool ourselves.

Adopt a Whole Program. *If you are to succeed in overcoming arthritis, you must adopt a complete program of health restoration.* Arthritis does not stand alone. Many patients complain of poor digestion, constipation, poor circulation. Many are victims of various nervous disorders. Many are overweight while others are wasted or emaciated. Overacidity of the stomach, a spastic colon, a malfunctioning gallbladder and/or other gastric or intestinal disorders often accompany the existing arthritis. All of these impairments must be corrected if the arthritis sufferer is to get well.

Oxygen Is Vital. Because the bloodstream is the carrier of oxygen, you can appreciate the effect of a healthy interrelationship between the circulation and the joints. To build a healthy bloodstream, the need for foods rich in iron and other essential minerals should be evident. A powerful source of iron is the apricot, as well as the green leafy vegetables. Iron serves to transport oxygen to the organs of the body. But always remember that to rebuild the bloodstream, all other essential food elements obtained from *live, vital, natural* foods are a *must*!

HOW LILA REGAINED HER HEALTH

Another patient whose case I shall describe here is Lila B. Lila, age 34, suffered from a severe form of arthritis affecting her whole back, the lumbo-sacral region of her spine as well as the upper part of her back and neck. Lila also suffered from constant attacks of indigestion, acute gallbladder seizures, recurring migraine headaches and extreme debility verging on collapse. She was greatly overweight.

To start with, I told her there would be no medicines, no antacid remedies for her indigestion and gallbladder pains. No sedatives or tranquilizers for her nerves. No pain relievers. These only disguised her pains in the past while her disorders continued to get worse.

Lila was put on the complete internal health-rebuilding regimen as described in this book. She followed this regimen consistently, and in about six to eight months all her pains and aches disappeared. Another gain that pleased her greatly was her new figure. When Lila started, she weighed 165 pounds. By the time she got well, she was a slim 125.

Lila had one weakness that had to be overcome. She ate heavily of acid-forming foods. These included meat, eggs and hard-fat-containing foods. She also had a tendency to overeat. She was taught to reduce, to eliminate the highly acid-forming foods, and to make sure not to overeat. She continued to make the needed changes in her diet and in her way of living and gradually grew into a normally healthy and vital woman.

Overacidity Weakens Bodily Functioning. Many meat and animal-source foods (including hard cheeses and eggs) create an acid-ash residue that irritates the pockets and internal parts of the bone structures as well as the vital body organs. In our plan to defeat arthritis, *the weakening of normal bodily functioning through overacidity must be checked. Overacidity plays an important role in the development of arithritis and causes a great deal of pain that can be avoided.*

Acid Producing Substances Must Be Avoided: Acetylsalicylic acid which is aspirin, acetic acid (vinegar), and various acid-forming foods such as the rich meats and grains, must be eliminated. Any foods made with or containing any of these acid-forming sources are TABOO. Also when purchasing foods, make it a practice to read available labels. Artificial substances or additives or preservatives that are listed on the packaged foods are often acid forming and increase the internal toxicity of the arthritis sufferer's body. Make sure that you use undenatured foods, and if possible prepare the meal in your own home. Coffee too is acid producing and its use should be discarded.

Neglected Ailments Lead to Arthritis. Neglected ailments such as recurring stomach pains, allergies, and pains and aches associated with changes of climate, often lead to a full-blown state of arithritis. Acute infectious diseases when treated by suppressive drugs, also predispose to the disease. The infectious disease is suppressed, but the toxic condition is not eliminated and eventually damage in the joints begins to show up.

A Change in Internal Body Chemistry:
the Key to Arthritis Control

Arthritis control calls for correction of whatever ailments or physical derangements exist in the body. To enjoy a life free from arthritis, we must restore normal bodily functioning and establish a state of equilibrium and balance.

A MIRACULOUS CHANGE IN 74-YEAR-OLD MRS. P.

The story of 74-year-old Mrs. Milda P. further illustrates why sufferers from arthritis who wish to get well must overcome not only their arthritis condition but also the various other disorders that are associated with it.

Mrs. P. suffered from a severe form of arthritis involving the right hip, knee and ankle, as well as pains and stiffness in her neck and extremely severe low back pains. Other ailments for which she had been treated for years were diabetes, high blood pressure, insomnia, and constipation.

For a person of her age she remembered well the many remedies that she had been taking during the years for her many pains and illnesses and was able to rattle their names off to me.

My first instruction was to discontinue all medication. Then I suggested that she take the hot epsom salt baths evenings before retiring and retire immediately after the bath.

Because of her diabetes, her diet had to be especially carefully planned. At first I instructed her to take no other food but a grapefruit for breakfast, a raw vegetable salad and one steamed vegetable for lunch, and a large raw vegetable salad with a small portion of lean fish or chicken or any other lean meat and one steamed vegetable for dinner. She was to use no salt or butter, and coffee, bread, soups and anything else not listed on the above menu, were to be eliminated.

Her blood was tested regularly for blood sugar, and this helped us to decide when other foods could be added. Gradually her diet was increased. For breakfast she could take half a grapefruit, to be followed one-half hour later by natural brown rice or buckwheat groats with raw grated apple and some skimmed milk. For lunch she had a raw vegetable salad with one baked potato and one steamed vegetable (no salt or butter). Also blueberries or peaches for dessert if she desired it. For dinner she was allowed a raw vegetable salad, a small portion of lean meat or fish and one steamed vegetable. She could also use two grapefruits and two apples a day. Later, since she missed her bread, she was allowed one slice of whole wheat toast daily.

She was instructed to do her deep breathing exercises and the milder leg exercises every morning and night. (I describe these exercises in a subsequent chapter.) She was told to take a nap or rest period after lunch, to make sure to get plenty of sleep, and to make an effort to move her bowels after each meal. Not to strain, but to make this a regular habit and keep at it until the desired results were attained.

What were the results after six months of this care? Her pains in her back, hips, knees, shoulders, and head have practically all disappeared. Without taking any drugs for her diabetes, her blood sugar is now completely under control even though her diet is rather liberal. She needs no pills to put her to sleep, she gets a good night's sleep every night. Her bowels are moving at least once and more often twice a day, and naturally, without help from laxatives. Her blood pressure too came down to near normal.

It did not take too long before Mrs. P. began to show highly significant improvement, but it is well to mention at this point that not all cases respond so rapidly. In some cases the various ailments may be more deeply rooted and/or the patient's body may be so greatly weakened and depleted that results can come only slowly and gradually. Furthermore, certain acute reactions often show up during the curative stage, and when they occur the patient must be prepared to accept them with equanimity and patience. Never permit yourself to be led astray when unexpected reactions occur. Reactions are part of the curative process, (I discuss this phase more fully in Chapter 14), and when during the curative period these reactions occur, you must realize what they imply and not let them frighten you. You must remember that the length of time it takes to get well depends to a great degree upon the extent of the damage in the body as well as upon the recuperative powers of the individual case. This most often determines whether results come quickly or whether more time is required before the body regains its health. But you can always be certain that in practically all cases, perseverance and patience will ultimately pay off in renewed health and well-being.

The Internal Cleansing Plan. In discussing internal cleanliness as a means of rebuilding the health of the arthritis sufferer, I am referring to something that is infinitely more important than what we have in mind when we discuss ordinary body cleanliness. Internal body cleanliness calls for measures that keep the bloodstream as well as all the internal organs and parts of the body in a physiologically heathy condition.

The aim is to build a clean and healthy bloodstream and to rebuild the functions of the kidneys, the colon, the lungs, the skin, and all other vital organs and tissues of the body so that by functioning efficiently they maintain the whole body in a state of good health. The nervous system must be strengthened and rebuilt. All the organs and tissues of the body have to be restored to normal functioning if we are to succeed in overcoming this body-wracking disease.

The Stream of Life. Blood, because of its importance to our body economy, is known as the "Stream of Life." To keep well, our joints must receive a constant supply of food and oxygen and must dispose of their waste products. When the blood is kept free from impurities and is able to circulate freely and efficiently, it supplies the joints with their nutrients and oxygen and carries off their impurities.

Living for one or even several days solely on fresh spring water when thirsty or hungry, or on fresh raw fruit and/or vegetable juices when desired, helps to promote the elimination of bodily toxins and lays the foundation for renewed health.

Corrective Elimination. When the bowels fail to function properly, retention of waste products in the colon results. This causes excessive fermentation and contributes to the accumulation of toxins in the systems. It also contributes to the building up of an impure bloodstream. To maintain corrective elimination, one glass of cold water flavored with a few drops of lemon juice every morning before taking any other food, is often recommended. And sip it slowly. Then wait for 30 minutes and drink one glass of orange juice, or as in the case of Mrs. P. eat your grapefruit. This often arouses the peristaltic waves of the colon and induces more normal elimination.

Improve Kidney Function and Relieve Arthritis. Kidneys that have become weakened through abuse or overwork cannot eliminate all the toxins that are carried to it by the blood, and this too leads to the retention of waste products in the system. The kidneys will react violently to harsh condiments, spices and artificial seasoning—whether applied by a shaker or cooked in the foods! To keep your kidneys healthy, do not abuse them with salt, pepper, sharp condiments, mustard, catsup, vinegar, so-called bitters, coffee, and the like. These irritate the filtering apparatuses of the kidneys.

Promote Healthy Skin Function. Your skin is an eliminative organ, and when it is unable to function properly, poisons are retained in the system, and this, too, leads to an impure bloodstream and general ill health. Restore healthy skin functioning with wholesome natural foods and sound natural hygienic care. This precludes artificial and concentrated sweets and starches. Exercises do much to rebuild the functioning of the skin. The hot baths are of great help, while a good friction rubdown with a brisk brush or a turkish towel brings a glowing feeling of warmth to the skin and promotes more normal functioning.

Healthy Lung Power. Air pollution is hazardous, so get out to the country for the weekends; go to the beaches, to the suburbs, or anywhere where you can breathe reasonably pure, clean air. Cleanse your lungs and they will be able to serve you better. It is by way of the lungs that we breathe in the pure, life-giving oxygen, the oxygen we need to neutralize toxic wastes in the system. The lungs also throw off bodily toxins in the form of a carbonic acid gas or carbon dioxide. Carbon dioxide is a normal by-product of metabolism and it has to be eliminated from the system. Poor or shallow breathing, or any impediment that slows down the elimination of these gaseous by-products is detrimental to health, and interferes with the rebuilding of the health of the arthritis sufferer.

Basic Ill Health Needs Treatment. When you see how essential the functions of the eliminative organs are, you immediately begin to understand how necessary it is to keep the internal organs of the body in a clean and healthy condition.

Care of Your Liver. Your liver plays a vital part in keeping the body healthy and clean, and sufferers from arthritis must not take anything into their system in the form of food, beverages, drugs, or chemicals that impair its functioning. The healthy liver performs an infinite number of vital metabolic functions. The liver is not only a vital digestive organ, it is also one of our most essential purification plants since it helps to neutralize the toxic substances that find their way into the system or that accumulate because of the breakdown or inefficient functioning of other vital organs.

Toxic Drugs and Chemicals Endanger the Liver. One of the reasons for insisting that those who suffer from arthritis stay away from all medication is because of its danger to the liver. I am thinking of a patient who after taking high blood pressure pills for several years come to me suffering from a severe cirrhosis of the liver with ascites or fluid in the abdomen. Fortunately the liver even when already badly damaged can often regenerate, and this patient after adopting my plan of care showed considerable improvement, but the danger to the liver when it has to neutralize toxic drugs or chemicals is very great.

To keep the system clean, the liver must do a great deal of work to neutralize toxic wastes and prepare them for elimination. This is why the liver must not be overtaxed by chemicals, drugs, or any of the unhealthy overprocessed foods or beverages. In a later chapter I discuss the various bodily reactions that arthritis sufferers often experience while the body eliminates its toxic wastes, and certain liver symptoms like yellow skin, or muddy complexion, yellowish tinge in the eyes or purplish lips; also headaches, dizziness, and tiredness indicate that the body is going through a detoxification process, and when this happens the liver usually carries the brunt of the burden. While these symptoms are often unpleasant and sometimes even frightening, they only show what is taking place and should serve as a warning that everything possible be done to bring about the needed detoxification as rapidly as possible. They show that the body is trying to rid itself of its waste products, but to be able to do this in a most efficient way, the liver must be kept in a healthy condition so that it can meet the challenge when it arises.

The Endocrine Glands Play a Vital Role in Fighting Arthritis. If the arthritis sufferer is to get well, the endocrine system, the glands that regulate the functions of all the organs of the body and maintain internal balance and equilibrium, must be rebuilt and strengthened.

Arthritis is caused in many ways. Wear and tear, old age, injury, infection, contribute to its onset. Also, most physicians who have made a close study of the subject, realize that a derangement in endocrine functioning is most often involved. This is why cortisone or its related hormones used in the treatment of the disease, while providing no lasting benefits, often provide dramatic relief. They artificially provide hormones that our own endocrine glands should naturally secrete, but are unable to do so. But since these artificially supplied hormones do not rebuild the functions of the exhausted or broken-down glands, they do not actually help to overcome the existing diseased or abnormal condition. What is even worse, since these artificially supplied hormones force the worn-out or deranged glands of the endocrine system to function at a more intensified rate and this at a time when they are already badly depleted, it ultimately leads only to further depletion. This causes only more damage and in time leads to more pain and greater crippling.

Injury as a Precipitating Factor. I refer on many occasions to the fact that physical injury can cause the onset of arthritis. A fall, a bruise, any form of injury, causes inflammation and/or congestion of a joint or joints, and often leaves them weakened and subject to the onset of arthritis.

Hot epsom salt baths followed by moist cold compresses applied to the injured part, are of great help in overcoming the weakening or damaging effects of a fall or injury. Complete rest or immobilization of the injured or weakened joint or joints is sometimes necessary, and the injured person must never overlook the benefits that are derived from good food and overall healthful care as an aid to the rebuilding of the injured part of the body.

How a Clean Lymphatic System Helps Defeat Arthritis. The lymphatic system comprises the channels and vessels that collect the tissue fluid known as lymph, and transport it back to the veins so that it re-enters the circulating blood. The lymphatic vessels have thin walls, and are associated with the capillaries. Like the smaller veins and the smaller arteries they join together into larger and larger lymphatic vessels which eventually lead into a large vessel known as the *thoracic duct*. This duct empties into one of the large veins near the heart. The lymph channels contain oval masses of lymphoid tissue called lymph nodes or lymph glands which play an important role in neutralizing toxins and in keeping the tissues of our body in a clean and healthy condition.

The fluid of the lymphatic system plays a vital part in keeping the body healthy. It bathes the cells, keeps them clean, and carries nutrients to them. It also carries off many toxic by-products. The lymphatic fluid contains dissolved proteins, fats, sugar, and everything else brought by the bloodstream and which the body requires. It also carries away from the cells waste products such as urea, uric acid, and white blood cells.

Urea and uric acid are toxic wastes. In many cases of arthritis such as gout, bursitis and low back pain, these toxic substances have accumulated in excessive amounts. They must be eliminated from the body.

Herbal teas help to flush from the kidneys some of these toxic substances. Many a coffee- and tea-drinking and cola-guzzling arthritic has experienced great relief when I put them on a natural herb-tea-drinking program. The bland herbs are Nature's gifts to man. They contain precious ingredients that neutralize internal acidity and help nullify the toxic materials that accumulate in the lymphatic system. Herb teas are available almost anywhere, but especially in health food shoppes throughout the country.

Correct Health Flaws. Inflamed tonsils, congested and swollen adenoids, enlarged glands in the neck, under the armpits, or in the groin are indications that toxins have accumulated in the system and that the glands are trying to neutralize them in an effort to protect our health. These health flaws must be corrected. Arthritis symptoms associated with such disorders also often clear up at the same time.

Decayed and abscessed teeth require attention. Wrong foods such as excessive sweets, refined and processed cereals, and other unwholesome foods and beverages, eat into the gums and teeth, often causing cavities and abscesses. I stress the need of sound dental care where this is necessary, but I also emphasize the need of adopting a sound health-building program since a continuation of the use of unhealthy foods and other unhealthy living habits only leads to more damage in the teeth and gums, and with it increases the damage to the entire organism. But beware of the doctor who tries to remove teeth wholesale on the assumption that this will correct your arthritis. This was a general practice years back, but the futility of this procedure has long been recognized.

There is no telling how many mouths have been ruined for life by this ruthless procedure in the mistaken belief that it would overcome this crippling disease.

Total Body Care Essential

What I said above explains why in the care of arthritis, we must not confine our hopes to remedies that provide mere relief of pain. We must adopt a program of care that promotes detoxification, purifies the bloodstream, and builds a clean and healthy body. This can only be done when a program of care based upon the use of natural foods and the aforementioned healthful practices is followed.

The chemistry of the body must be restored to its normal condition. The nervous system must be strengthened and rebuilt. Digestive and eliminative disorders must be overcome. The glands and organs whose functions have become impaired must be rehabilitated. This can in most instances be accomplished only when pain-relieving drugs are discontinued and a program of living and care as outlined in this book is followed.

THE PROGRAM THAT HEALED A "HOPELESS" CASE

It was saddening to look at Mr. Lucien A. when he first came in for treatment. He was bent over, heavy, and appeared very much older than his middle 40's. He suffered from a difficult type of arthritis which handicapped him greatly. Severe shoulder and neck pains caused spasms and a great deal of pain when, while driving or backing out from his garage, he had to turn his head.

X rays disclosed severe rheumatic and arthritic deformities. They showed many arthritis "spurs" which cut into the soft flesh and caused gripping pains. He was in despair when he applied for help, and noting his overall arthritis condition I began to wonder if he could be helped. His family physician told him that he would have to learn to live with his illness, but he was not ready to accept this decision and came to find out what he could do so that he could be helped.

My First Advice. After a thorough examination, I told him that since his condition had been allowed to progress for many years, it would take an extensive period of time before the arthritis in his back could be reversed, and that he would not accomplish very much unless he agreed to adhere faithfully to the program that I would outline for him.

He wanted to know how long it would take before he would get better, but nobody can really say with any certainty. Some cases show a great deal of improvement in four to six months—while cases of long standing and with intensive damage may require a year or two or even longer before their arthritis is brought under complete control.

Diet Approach. Lucien was put on a natural diet—steamed vegetables with *no* seasoning of any sort, raw vegetable salad, fruit, cottage cheese and baked potatoes. Because he craved some seasoning, he was allowed a small amount of diced onion and lemon juice on his salad. As for salad oils, small amounts of soybean oil or corn oil were allowed. He could also use a moderate portion of avocado with his raw vegetables or raw fruits. No sugar. No salt. No condiments. No butter. No coffee. No tea. Fresh fruit or vegetable juices were allowed but no milk, and none of the commercial soft drinks. He was told to abstain from sweets, cookies, candies and cakes. These are loaded with "empty calories" and contain additives which infiltrate the bloodstream and leave waste deposits that tend to accumulate in the tissues.

Protein from Non-meat Sources. Meat was restricted because it is an acid-forming food. The bloodstream of an arthritis sufferer is often overladen with acid, so further burdening is only an added hardship. Protein was to come from cottage cheese. Twice a week, lean poultry or lean fish could be eaten. A sparse amount of very lean broiled meat could be included at the end of the second week. (It might be mentioned that chicken and fish had to be broiled. NO fried foods of any sort.)

Exercises and Warmth. Lucien was given home exercises to perform, and also sunlamp treatments. He followed a wide variety of different types of exercises designed to relieve his kinked up muscles and skeletal structures. Gradually, these treatments eased congestion. Slowly, he began to feel better.

First Signs of Recovery. His skin cleared up. (His skin had shown many blemishes and was badly irritated.) A fungus infection of his feet known as athlete's foot was overcome. There was also a clearing up of his sinus condition; a notable absence of colds which in the past interrupted his activities periodically. He would take daily naps and then have a good night's sleep. He would awaken refreshed and ready for his working schedule. His varicose veins improved. The numbness of his legs and feet, resulting from poor circulation, now all but vanished. He could even return to skiing again. Best of all, his taste buds became keener, more alive. He began to enjoy natural foods with gourmet gusto.

After almost a year of intensive care, Lucien A. continues on with his program. He has a general schedule of exercises about five minutes in the morning and five minutes in the evening. He no longer has the headaches which often plagued him in previous years. He suffered from pyorrhea before he came to me and his dentist confirmed that his gums had greatly improved. There was just one exception to his natural plan when he underwent a hernia operation and the removal of a polyp from his abdomen. He spent a week or two in the hospital and was given the usual dose of sedatives. Otherwise, Nature has helped restore him to health and arthritic freedom. Now he is a living example of what this type of care can do for sufferers from arthritis.

HOW INTERNAL MALFUNCTIONING LEADS TO ARTHRITIS

When she was 54, Sadie G. felt the first warning signs of arthritis. Her joints swelled. Her knees were hot to the touch. She was bedridden. Cortisone distorted her face and gave it a moon-like appearance. She found out she had congestive heart failure and her blood pressure was over 200. Her kidneys were unable to function, and when she was rushed to the hospital she was told that she had internal bleeding. Mrs. G. was given blood transfusions and put under oxygen for a few weeks.

Nothing seemed to relieve her arthritis. She lived, but when she came home, she was an invalid. That was how she was brought to us and placed under Dr. Stanley Weinsier's and my supervision. She came in a wheelchair. X rays of Mrs. G. showed that she suffered not only from a complicated arthritis condition, but also from a greatly enlarged heart.

We corrected her diet. She was first given only small amounts of fruit, small raw vegetable salads and baked potatoes. She was put on a partial fast. Then she was given more fruits, more vegetables and brown rice. Slowly, her medications were discontinued. A plan of exercises, short walks, and a daily whirlpool bath, augmented her restoration to health.

For nineteen weeks, she underwent this natural therapy until she was able to knit and use her arms and legs. When she returned home, her heart was normal in size. She was ready to do her own housework, even entertain. It took altogether about three years before her health was completely rebuilt. Recently she was examined by the physician who x-rayed her joints when she first came to us for treatment, and he was amazed to find that the massive calcium deposits in the knees and other joints had completely disappeared. From a bedridden invalid, she had become a useful human being.

Saved from the Surgeon's Knife. I will always remember Mrs. Margaret W., who suffered from a severe form of arthritis, with pains all over her body. Going from doctor to doctor she received all kinds of treatments, including diathermy, X rays and injections, but without results. Then she went to a doctor who told her that her X rays showed calcium deposits in her shoulders and that she required surgery. He said he would have to operate and "scrape the bones." "I felt like lightning hit me. How could they scrape my bones when I had pains all through my body. That was the last time I saw that doctor," Mrs. W. explained.

She heard about my type of care and came to see whether I could help her. I placed her on an internal housecleaning program as well as special fasting days. Fasting is an ancient remedy that detoxifies the body and helps cleanse the tissues and cells of their accumulated waste products. At first Margaret W. was placed on a short fast. Then she was placed on a careful eating plan with special emphasis on shredded or grated raw vegetables.

Here is a typical arthritis diet such as Mrs. W. followed:

Breakfast: Orange juice, small bowl of oatmeal or brown rice, prunes, skimmed milk.

Mid-morning: A glass of freshly squeezed carrot-celery-parsley juice.

Lunch: One small apple, one celery stalk, one small carrot, all grated fine with two dates cut up and a spoonful of finely ground nuts or cottage cheese or a baked potato.

Supper: Meat in moderation. Broiled chicken or fish. Occasionally, the meat dish could be a small portion of steak. (Once a week, fish fillet broiled was permitted.) In place of fish or meat she was encouraged to use a baked potato several times a week. She was also to use a raw vegetable salad with the meal and could also use one steamed vegetable and a fruit for dessert if still hungry.

Must Food. A large mixed green salad every single day of the year. It must be a salad of RAW vegetables.

This kind of diet plus corrective physical exercises, controlled sunbathing which stimulates the formation of Vitamin D beneath the surface of the skin, and sufficient physical rest, all help Nature to bring about the needed rebuilding.

Margaret W. recovered completely from her ailment. What's more she was spared surgery. This was over 20 years ago. Now past 70 and as spry as ever, she exercises daily, works in her garden, and is happy that she has learned how to continue to stay well.

Health Begins with a Return to Rational Living. Because arthritis is usually the result of basic ill health, treatment is planned along lines that rebuild the health of the entire body. This means natural foods, a regulated program of exercises, restoration of the functions of all the organs and glands that need rebuilding. The entire body must receive the care it needs to bring about internal purification and normal functioning.

Principles Outlined in This Chapter

1. Arthritis is often initiated when health impairment strikes other parts of the body.
2. Rebuild health from the inside.
3. Eliminate impurities with corrective breathing techniques and other body-purifying care.
4. Excess acid-forming foods should be greatly restricted or completely eliminated.
5. Your liver, your colon, your glands, your lymphatic system, need internal cleansing and rebuilding to help defeat arthritis.
6. Many "hopeless" cases were restored to complete recovery by following a physiologically adequate diet and by adhering to a natural *health-building program*.
7. Arthritis sufferers must not expect to get well over night. Time, patience, and perseverance are required. You must persist in following this health-building program if you are to attain the desired benefits.

3

HOW TO RECOGNIZE AND
CARE FOR THE MAJOR TYPES
OF ARTHRITIS

Many cases of debility could be prevented if arthritis were to be recognized in its early stages. The sooner corrective measures are initiated, the better the chance for a more thorough recovery. Arthritis is the most common of all causes of physical disability —so very common, in fact, that there are few families in which some member has not felt its disabling effects.

Neglect May Increase Arthritis. Neglect is your worst enemy in the elimination of arthritis. Early, continuing health care is your greatest asset. Care does not mean taking pain-relieving drugs but rebuilding the health of the whole body. Early awareness of what you must do to counteract this crippling disease before it takes firm root in your body can save much suffering and protect you against many needless and avoidable heartaches. Care in the early stages of the disease will shield you against its deeper inroads and make correction so much easier.

Avoid Drugs. When you are able to nip arthritis in the bud, you prevent it from getting worse and protect yourself against the temptation of taking drugs. Salicylates and aspirins introduce toxic factors in the blood and lymph systems, and when these factors accumulate in the body they often aggravate rather than help to combat the condition.

Gold salts, phenylbutazone and many other remedies are prescribed for arthritis pains, but they certainly don't cure the dis-

51

ease. A physician may also use hormones, those tongue-twisting steroids such as cortisone, prednisone or prednisolene. In some cases, even very small doses of these drugs can produce serious side effects. None of these drugs cures. They only disguise the disease and when the drugs are discontinued, the symptoms return and often in a much more severe form.

In advanced arthritis cases, the intense pains are usually accompanied by stiffness and swelling. My experience with thousands of patients proved that when the early warnings of arthritis are recognized and the program of care that I am presenting in this book is followed, the disease is usually stopped from progressing, and then recovery begins.

Is This Happening to You?

1. When you bend over, do you experience a knife-like pain in your lower back?

2. When you rotate your wrists do you hear them "pop"? When you twist your shoulders do you hear them "cracking and creaking"?

3. When you turn your head or bend it backward looking at the ceiling, do you hear your neck snap?

4. At night do you find it difficult to turn around freely in bed?

5. Do you experience considerable stiffness in joints which normally should be flexible; for example, your elbows, your shoulders, your knees, your ankles? You may not realize it, but the lining in your joints has become defective and fails to provide the necessary lubrication.

6. Do you feel numbing aches in the region of your joints, especially after you have done an average amount of work?

7. Do you suffer from recurring backaches or recurring pains shifting from one joint to another?

8. Do you feel chilling sensations in your limbs, numbness, other signs of poor circulation? Do you look pale and anemic?

9. After a night's rest do you feel tired and weary with pains showing up in your back or limbs?

10. Do climatic changes, such as change of weather before rain, cause pains and aches in your limbs?

How Early Recognition Can Lead to Recovery. Watch for these early warning signs listed above and protect yourself accordingly. When you are able to recognize these early arthritis symptoms or the other disturbances that often precede the onset of arthritis, correct them immediately and prevent them from growing into a more serious problem. Recognition is a prime factor in defeating arthritis before it takes firm root. It means that you can strike back while the disease is still in its formative stages and deterioration of the bones and other tissues of the joints has not yet set in.

The plan that helps arthritis patients in its early stages includes rest and relaxation. The patient must avoid fatigue and worry. A well planned set of exercises is of great help and the use of all-natural nourishing foods to maintain the body in good health is important. Extra pounds have to be melted away because overweight aggravates arthritis by placing an unnecessary strain on the joints. Overweight may also mean that there is an overall metabolic disorder that must be corrected by proper physical care as well as a healthful diet plan.

Most important, your own positive attitude is of great help in overcoming arthritis; often it is the true "miracle drug," since a hopeful attitude encourages you to follow this program faithfully and helps you get well faster. Your mental attitude often determines whether you become an invalid and a hopeless burden to family and friends, or whether you get well and continue as an active and useful member of your family and the community.

And as I stated previously, the sooner you give yourself the care you need, the better are your chances for recovery. Also by striking at arthritis before you give it a chance to gain firm roots, you avoid the temptation of turning to pain-relieving drugs and narcotics with their harmful side effects.

What Is Arthritis? In brief, arthritis (arth = joint, itis = inflammation) is a condition that may appear from time to time in one's life as a mild or occasional discomfort; or it increases relentlessly to complete crippling and invalidism.

In its chronic state it is usually a slow crippling disease of the joints. In the earlier stages, the pains are not always constant; they often come and go, but when of long standing, permanent injury in the joints ultimately sets in. Hands, feet and other joints of the body, may then become gnarled and crippled for life.

How It Begins. Arthritis is a disease that often strikes because of a disturbance in body metabolism, or arises as a result of prolonged abuse or abnormal wear and tear of the joints. It develops also as an aftermath of injury or trauma. Earlier acute illnesses when improperly treated often plant the seed for this disease in children as well as in adults. The presence of abscessed teeth and tonsils, and similar "focal" or "local" infections may precede the onset of this crippling disease. A sudden injury such as a fall, a sprain, a fracture, or laceration, or any infectious disease when neglected or treated the wrong way, can leave a defect which later develops into arthritis. Frequently, a shock to the nerves, tension over a prolonged period of time, arteriosclerotic changes in the body, all set up chain reactions that ultimately form different types of arthritis.

Arthritis Often Mistaken for Other Rheumatic Disorder. Because arthritis belongs to the "rheumatic family," its beginnings are often mistaken for one of its related diseases such as lumbago, neuritis, or sciatica. Arthritis is often classified under a variety of names, but whether it is called by one name or another we must always bear in mind that all arthritic and rheumatic diseases arise as a result of the same or similar health-deteriorating influences and can only be corrected through sound systemic care applied in conformity with sound natural healing principles. This approach is applicable in all cases of arthritis, those that develop slowly and insidiously as well as those that set in abruptly and that are accompanied by high fever or sudden intense pains. We must never forget that the factors that have made this disease flare up suddenly, have most often been laying the foundation for its eruption for a long time.

In most cases though, the first symptoms may be so fleeting and superficial that they are often disregarded. This is a mistake, since

these warning signals, if heeded in time could save untold agony.
A feeling of numbness or stiffness, creaking and cracking of the
joints, occasional twinges, cold clammy hands and feet, a burning sensation in the feet, or such peculiar sensations as that of
ants crawling under the skin, should serve as a warning that something is wrong and that it must not be neglected.

The Changes in the Joints

Arthritis is a disease of the joints, affecting the bones that make
up the joint as well as its soft and semi-soft tissues. The ends of
the bones that meet to make up the joint are covered by a semi-
soft elastic substance which in common parlance is known as the
gristle but in medical language is known as the cartilage. The
cartilage cushions the joint and minimizes friction and strain.
The inner surface of the joint cavity is covered by a lining known
as the synovial membrane which secrets a light, yellowish, semi-
liquid gelatinous substance to keep the joint lubricated and protect it against jarring or shock.

What Happens to the Joint?

When increasing amounts of waste products accumulating in
the system interfere with the supply of nutrition and oxygen to
the joint or impair its ability to rid itself of its waste products, a
certain amount of damage ultimately begins to show up in the
joints and this is how arthritis develops. The cartilage, the substance that protects the interlocked bones against undue friction
and strain, in time becomes brittle and hardened, gradually losing
its pliability and in the later stages often wastes away completely.
The synovial membrane that secretes the protective synovial fluid
also becomes impaired. At first it may pour out more of the lubri-
cating fluid that is needed to keep the joint in a healthy condition
but later its ability to secrete the needed lubrication diminishes,
and in time even dries up completely.

There are a great many other changes that take place. The joint
becomes infiltrated with calcium and becomes thickened and enlarged while the bones that make up the joint often become irregular, rough, jagged, or overgrown with bony deposits or spurs.

These changes impair the ability of the joint to function freely and cause untold suffering.

Osteoporosis a Serious Health Problem

As I pointed out before, arthritis is a disorder of metabolism. In the earlier stages of the disease too much calcium accumulates in the joints while in the more advanced stages, essential minerals are often leached out from the bones and then we have the condition known as osteoporosis. When too much calcium accumulates the joint thickens and enlarges and this often causes a great deal of pain and crippling while when osteoporosis sets in the bones become fragile or weakened and break easily. Fragile or weakened bones often shift their position or fracture and this often causes pressure on the adjacent tissues and often even leads to a certain amount of paralysis.

Irritating Toxins

When irritating toxins settle in the shoulder joint, a painful inflammation known as bursitis sets in. These toxic by-products accumulating in the lower back cause the condition known as lumbago or arthritis. A rheumatic inflammation of the muscles with or without pain is called myalgia, myositis, fibrositis, or muscular rheumatism. Nerve pains are known as neuritis or neuralgia. A sciatic nerve inflammation shows up as sciatica or sciatic rheumatism.

Toxins Are to Blame

Except when caused by an injury or some mechanical interference causing local pressure on nerves, arthritis is the result of stagnation or poisoning caused by the toxins retained in the body. Neglect or failure to treat these conditions when they first begin to show up by following a thorough detoxification and health-rebuilding program ultimately leads to the development of the more severe forms of arthritis. In the great majority of cases it is the accumulation of irritating toxins that leads to an impairment in body metabolism and that ultimately gives rise to the onset of this disease.

Strike the Disease at the Source

The *causes* of arthritis must be eradicated. This includes purifying the blood stream and throwing off the toxins that have accumulated in the tissues. The blood and the tissues must be kept in a clean and healthy condition since this helps to provide the joints with the nutrients and oxygen they need to get them well and keep them well.

Rheumatoid Arthritis

This type of arthritis originates from disturbances which undermine the health of the body as a whole and is most debilitating. It starts with an inflammation of the synovial membrane, the lining that provides the lubrication for the joint, but then spreads to the other parts of the joint such as the cartilage, the tendons, the ligaments, the muscles and the bones. In time it leads to considerable deformity and crippling.

How Rheumatoid Arthritis Starts. It develops gradually and insidiously. There may be sudden fever, or weakness and pains in many joints. The joints of the fingers, wrists, knees, and feet become swollen and tender. There is great debility. Pains and tenderness are usually most pronounced in the morning upon awaking, but lessen with the day's activities. Overstrain or tension often leads to much pain the day after. Muscle spasms and joint swellings are often part of the picture.

As the disease continues to develop, joint destruction increases. Destruction of the cartilage with a narrowing of the joint space takes place. Ankylosis or permanent stiffening of the joints, continuous pains, as well as muscular shrinkage and wastage make their appearance in the more advanced stages of this type of arthritis.

Serious Consequences. In the more severe cases, the heart may become involved although, as a rule, much less often than in rheumatic fever and usually in less intense form. Some of these cases are accompanied by a difficult and sometimes intractable skin disease known as psoriasis. In other cases serious eye problems may arise. Iritis, an inflammation of one of the membranes in the eyeball accompanied by pain and swelling, sometimes accompanies this type of arthritis.

Rheumatoid arthritis is three times more common among women than among men. Although the whole body is usually affected, the joints suffer most. Usually the smaller joints are affected first—those of the fingers as a rule. Whether the pain comes on suddenly or slowly by "twinges," swelling and discomfort in these joints may come and go for years. They appear first in one part of the body, then in other parts.

Each recurring attack is more severe and more incapacitating. Eventually, the joints become permanently damaged causing limitation of motion and sometimes complete invalidism.

Since this type of arthritis is of a constitutional nature and originates from disturbances that affect the body as a whole, it is fallacious to look for a remedy that provides mere relief of the existing joint pains. It can only be overcome when the health of the entire body is rebuilt.

From Sciatica to Crippling Arthritis and Then Turning to Nature for a Cure

How does natural healing help in rheumatoid arthritis? Let us see what it has done for Molly F. For three years, Molly F. suffered from arthritis, lumbago, sciatica, neuritis and neuralgia. It began with sciatica of the left leg. When Mrs. F. tried to get out of bed one morning, she was seized with a knife-like pain. She had spent a week in bed with the grippe and high fever. She could barely move her lower body. When she stooped to pick up something, she couldn't straighten up. Sharp, stabbing pains seized the lower part of her back. It was recurrent: it disappeared but then suddenly returned. Nightly, the stabbing pains were most distressing and she would cry aloud. She was not ashamed to say she often cried herself to a nervous sleep.

(Sciatica is a form of neuritis of the sciatic nerve causing excruciating pain along the course of this nerve, the largest nerve in the body which runs down the back of the thigh and into the leg).

The pain that radiated into her left leg became progressively worse, and then settled down to a persistent throb like a dull toothache. Mrs. F. could sit only on one side. She took salicylates and codeine but with no improvement. There were times when her knee was so stiff and painful she had to drag her leg when walking.

Gradually, the insidious internal "infection" spread to other joints. Her arms ached, her fingers were painful. She went to a doctor who gave her all kinds of injections, but this led to swelling as well as accompanying redness and soreness. The pain continued. Her condition became progressively worse and at the age of 36, she could see nothing but a dreary and hopeless future. She could no longer even play the piano which she had always loved. She could see nothing but sickness, pain and hopelessness ahead of her.

When Mrs. F. came to see me, she told me how she had had several healthy teeth extracted because of the pains in her jaw. She had taken so much codeine, it began to lose its effect. She was constantly wracked with pain. Mrs. F. broke into an uncontrollable crying spell when she told me that she was afraid she would never again be well.

I placed her first on a fruit juice and vegetable juice diet. Then we followed with a wholesome vegetable diet. No meats. No animal-source foods. She took daily hot salt baths. She discontinued all of her medicines. She was trained to control her emotions, to develop a calm outlook, to relax.

It took seven months of this program before the pains subsided, and by then she was on the road to recovery. The secret, if any, is that her arthritis and sciatica were not *individually* treated to the exclusion of the rest of her body. It is only by treating the whole body that nature can truly heal. I might also add that Mrs. F. suffered from a severe gallbladder condition, and that after regaining her health she never again experienced a pain or an ache in the gallbladder region.

A Case of Rheumatoid Arthritis Healed

Lillian M. was in her early 40's when she developed rheumatoid arthritis. She was under the care of many doctors and received all kinds of injections—gold injections and others which made her very ill. A renowned orthopedic physician also operated on her foot and this only made her more sick. As time went on her pains traveled to other parts of her body and her hands became so swollen and painful that she could neither dress herself nor use them to even cut her food and eat properly. Going from one doctor to another and constantly continuing to get worse, she finally lost all hope of ever getting well and thought that she was doomed to a state of permanent invalidism.

At the recommendation of a friend she decided to place herself under my care. This was in May and by July she showed such remarkable improvement that it was almost unbelievable. Her swellings and her pains had practically all cleared up.

How was Mrs. M. helped? Quite simple. She discontinued all drugs. She adopted the plan of care that I am presenting in this book and followed it faithfully. I placed her on repeated fruit juice diets, outlined a well regulated dietary plan, recommended the daily epsom salt baths, and insisted that she do her exercises daily and get an abundance of sleep and rest.

Not all cases get well as quickly as Mrs. M. Mrs. F.'s case took much longer. The time it takes for these patients to get well depends to a great degree upon the existing degree of damage as well as upon the recuperative powers of the body. However, whether the sufferer from this type of arthritis gets well quickly or more time is required before the desired help is attained, it is well to realize that only when you work with the forces of nature are lasting benefits derived.

Osteoarthritis

This type of arthritis is also known as degenerative arthritis, degenerative joint disease, and hypertropic arthritis. It begins as a splintering and disintegration of the cartilage which covers the ends of the bones where they join to form a joint. As the cartilage wears away or becomes hardened and brittle, the underlying bone is exposed causing friction and pain upon movement. The gliding surfaces of the smooth normal cartilage are slowly replaced by hardening and thickening bone.

Frequently, this leads to bony overgrowths which cause pain and pressure at the end of the joints or its adjacent tendons and ligaments. The joints now become limited in motion because of thickening, pressure and pain. As the condition progresses other destructive changes and ultimate crippling set in.

Symptoms. Movement of the affected joints may be accompanied by a sensation of grating or crunching. Frequently there is audible cracking, creaking, or snapping. The affected joints may be touch-tender. Swelling, redness and an increase of heat in the joint often accompany these changes. In its early stages, this type of arthritis is usually not recognizable because the person may be able to move the joints, while the thickening and destruction of the cartilage and the other tissues slowly but steadily continue. There is gradual loss of the elasticity of the cartilage, and the adjoining bones fail to get the necessary protection. Eventually, when the arthritis has progressed to a dangerous state, the range of movement becomes greatly impaired. In time an overgrowth of bone develops and the joint is in danger of becoming completely ossified.

Which Joints Become Distorted by Osteoarthritis? Almost any bodily joint, but most frequently those joints which bear the greater part of body weight are distorted; that is, the spine, the hips, and the knees. Women seem to be afflicted in the end joints of their fingers. The appearance is that of a firm bony thickening which gives a knobby or gnarled appearance. These knobby, thickened joints are known as Herberdon's Nodes.

Finger Deformities. The enlargement of the finger joints may be the first signs that arthritis is present. Sometimes no other signs of arthritis are present, but their presence should be sufficient warning that arthritis is developing. In other cases these finger deformities are accompanied by overall bodily pains throughout the back, hips and legs. Sometimes headaches, dizziness, earaches, twitching, and neck distortions are felt. There are a variety of other disorders involving the head and the face.

Osteoarthritis as Caused by Unhealthy Living. Osteoarthritis as well as all other forms of arthritis is most often the outgrowth of impaired bodily functioning. Because of unhealthy living habits, bodily health begins to break down. When the circulation to the joints becomes impaired they fail to receive the nutrients and the oxygen they need to keep them healthy and they are unable to dispose of their toxic waste products. This impairs their functioning and leads to stagnation and congestion. Various destructive changes then begin to set in.

Excess calcium deposits in and around the joints and causes them to enlarge or thicken. Or osteoporosis develops; the bones become rarified or porous. Or some bones thicken while others become porous and weakened. These changes often set in, *not* because of a lack of calcium or too much calcium, but because the body is not in condition to utilize the calcium in the body. When the bones become hardened and thickened they cause a great deal of pain and often crippling. When they become porous or rarified they yield easily to pressure and often fracture. This causes numbness, chronic weakness, and often even paralysis.

Injuries Often Responsible. Overstrain of the weight-bearing joints or actual injury often leads to this form of arthritis. The arthritis may show up in the joint that has been abused or injured, but sometimes the joint on the opposite side now carrying an added burden may develop arthritis.

Osteoarthritis Causes Other Disorders. I pointed out earlier that before arthritis develops, many disorders precede its onset. In turn, this disease also gives rise to other disorders. When it settles in the spine it affects the spinal nerves, and the organs whose functions are controlled by these nerves become irritated. This leads not only to pain and stiffness in the back, it also causes a derangement in the functioning of the organs and tissues which are controlled by these nerves.

This is why osteoarthritis in the neck's upper part may cause pain to spread over the back of the skull and produce headaches. When it strikes the lower part of the neck, the pain spreads into the shoulder, then down into the arm and forearm and into the hands and fingers.

When it settles in the region between the shoulder blades it may cause pain to spread around the sides of the body to the chest cage, the heart, and the stomach region.

When the hip joints become affected, the pain shows up in a deep spasm in the buttocks, the groin, or over the outer surface of the hips. The pain may also spread to the thighs and the knees. Sometimes, pain felt in the knees may be the only symptom of osteoarthritis actually located in the hip joints. Deep abdominal pains and spasms may also be caused this way. Acute sciatic attacks often originate from pressure exerted by arthritis on the sciatic nerve.

How Weight Reduction Helped Mrs. H.

A case of osteoarthritis that illustrates what can be accomplished in this type of arthritis is the one of Florence H., age 60. Her back, her neck, her hips and her knees were already badly deformed when she came to see me and she also suffered from high blood pressure. She was also greatly overweight. After following a well regulated diet and a corrective exercise program for several months, and making all the other necessary adjustments, the arthritis in her joints cleared up almost entirely. She regained complete flexibility of the knees and hips, was able to move her neck freely and became entirely pain-free.

She also reduced her weight considerably. When she started she weighed 178 pounds but by the time she completed her visits with me she was a slim 148 and her blood pressure was 146/86.

In getting her started I prepared the following set of exercises which she was to do twice daily in addition to the diet and the bathing regimen that made up part of her health-rebuilding program.

1. She was to begin with the mild leg raising exercises. Without bending her knees, she was to raise first one leg three times, as high as she could reach and then lower it. Then she was to repeat the same exercise with the other leg, and then with both legs.

2. Then I suggested that she adopt a deep breathing exercise schedule. Keeping her mouth closed, she was to breathe in and out slowly and deeply, first through both nostrils, and then while blocking one nostril with her finger, breathe in and out through the other nostril, doing this for both nostrils. She was to do this five times each morning and night.

Finally, she was instructed to carry out a series of neck exercises. She was to rotate her head slowly first to one side, then to the other and repeat this exercise five times. Then she was to bend her head first to one side, then to the other side five times. These exercises are fully explained in Chapter 9.

It should not be necessary to tell how elated Mrs. H. was when her pains started to diminish. At last she knew that she was on the road to recovery. Mrs. H's loss of weight also pleased her since this made her look much younger and healthier.

Gouty Arthritis

Like other forms of arthritis, gout is a disease of the entire body, even though most of the suffering is felt in the joints. Hence, the secret of success in getting the gouty arthritis sufferer well is in rebuilding the health of the whole body. In acute gout the pains are sharp and the joints are extremely inflamed and painful. The big toe usually suffers most but other joints also often suffer. Most sufferers from this disease are men.

What Causes Gout? Actually, gout is a defect in the body's chemistry. There is an increase of uric acid in the system and this is caused not merely by wrong food or too much food, but by a defect in body metabolism. Some mistakenly assume that the accumulation of an excess of uric acid causes gout but actually the accumulation of the uric acid and the gout are caused by the same disorder, a derangement in body metabolism. This metabolic abnormality causes an increased accumulation or uric acid in the tissues and in the blood. Normally, uric acid is excreted by the kidneys, but erroneous living habits cause a disturbance in bodily functioning and in uric acid metabolism. Uric acid crystals are then deposited in the cartilages, chiefly found at the ends of the bones where they form the smooth surfaces of the joints.

Gouty arthritis, in its advanced stages, is the result of a toxic irritation set up around the joints by these crystals. An inflammatory reaction to the uric acid crystals brings on an acute attack of gout. The kidneys can secrete only a certain amount of the uric acid crystals that accumulate in the body. The rest is accumulated in the tissues, and when they deposit in the joints, gouty arthritis ultimately develops.

Symptoms Increase. Gradually, these sandy and hardened crystal-like deposits accumulate, forming large masses of "tophi" or chalky salts of uric acid. They may appear around almost any joint, but most commonly around the big toe and also on the external ear, the cartilages, the bones, and the tendons. The deposits are painless. But joint inflammation is painful, and the inflammation arises because the joints are trying to get rid of the "foreign" substance, a substance that does not belong there. Furthermore, the kidneys may be damaged and uric acid kidney stones may form.

Wrong Living. Gout is caused by wrong or high living. Overindulgence in unnatural foods and alcohol may bring on an acute attack or hasten the development of tophi. Overweight makes the disease more severe and more difficult to control.

Early Signs. An acute attack of gout may set in suddenly, and often in the middle of the night. The victim awakens with a sharp pain. Afterwards, there are frequent strikes of pain. There is a rapid increase in pain, swelling, redness, and heat in the joints which become agonizingly painful and tender.

The skin around the inflamed joint becomes shiny, taut and purplish. The joints may enlarge to as much as the size of a golf ball, and weakness and low fever may accompany the condition.

The first attack may last for less than an hour. Or it may go on for several days or weeks. When neglected or what is even worse, when treated by pain-deadening drugs, it ultimately progresses to a chronic deforming stage. Large masses of toxic uric acid salts are deposited around and in the joints, eventually damaging them.

Drugs May Trigger Attack. While gout is often caused by unwholesome acid-building foods, drugs and injections such as liver and penicillin shots may also start an attack. Some diuretics, by interfering with the kidney's excretion of uric acid, may precipitate an acute attack. This explains why these offending substances or drugs must be avoided, why a healthful, alkaline-building dietary program is essential, and why the overall health of the body must be rebuilt.

While other influences besides food contribute to the development of gout or gouty arthritis, the type of food eaten and how the body can handle it, plays a most important role. Rich, highly concentrated acid-producing foods, as well as highly processed and refined foods and beverages may cause a defect in metabolism and lead to the accumulation of uric acid crystals. Again, I must emphasize the importance of keeping the organs of digestion-assimilation-elimination in good working order and in a state of balance.

Internal Sludge. One of the most frightening cases of gout I have ever seen was that of a young, extremely heavy man in whom a great many of his joints were badly damaged by this disease. Not only were his gouty joints badly deformed, his hands, fingers, knees and hips had become immensely enlarged and thickened and many of his greatly enlarged and deformed joints showed large gaping wounds from which chalky uric acid crystals were being discharged.

His finger joints were so badly misshapen and enlarged in size that each single joint looked almost like a tennis ball.

During all my years of practice I have never come across a similar case, and this was one of the few cases of arthritis that I have seen in my practice where I felt that the destructive changes had progressed too far for me to be able to help him. This man must have suffered a great deal of agonizing pain during the many years that he had suffered from this disease and I have often wondered how much misery he could have avoided had he during the earlier stages of his illness found his way to the type of care that I am discussing in this book.

The average case of gouty arthritis may be difficult, but with good care and patience it usually responds and most often can be wholly corrected. Acute flare-ups may have to be expected while the body is trying to cleanse itself of the uric acid crystals that have accumulated in the joint or joints. It is actually during these acute stages when the joints become red, inflamed, angry looking and greatly enlarged that the uric acid crystals are being cleaned out. The inflammation gradually subsides, but acute reactions tend to recur and the condition ultimately grows more chronic unless a plan of care that helps to correct the disordered metabolism is adopted.

Foods and Beverages on the Forbidden List. Sufferers from gouty arthritis must make sure to avoid anchovies, clams, fish roe, scallops, shellfish and shrimp. They should omit brains, duck, goose, kidneys, liver, pork, sausage, scrapple, squab, sweetbread and tongue. Gravies, meat soups, meat extracts, alcohol, coffee and cola drinks must also be excluded. Sugars, cake, pastry, ice cream, sharp spices and condiments are also taboo. These foods and beverages cause an increase in uric acid and therefore must be eliminated.

But this is only part of the story. Sufferers from gout or gouty arthritis must plan a complete change in their foods and dietary habits and must make all the adjustments in their way of living that help uproot the existing gouty disorder and that rebuild the overall functioning of the whole body. This ultimately overcomes the tendency to produce and accumulate excessive amounts of uric acid in the system and helps to eradicate the disease.

Once you have become aware that this or any other form of arthritis is getting hold of you, stop neglecting yourself! Start following a health-building program in accordance with the principles outlined in this book. Do not procrastinate, do not delay, and do not delude yourself by thinking that remedies that suppress the acute attack can get you well, for this is only the road to more disease, greater suffering, and ultimately leads only to a more intensified or chronic form of gouty arthritis.

Many are the forms of arthritis. When we recognize the harmful effects of retained internal wastes and become aware of the damage they do to the bones and related tissues, we can well understand how a program that detoxifies the system, builds a clean, healthy bloodstream and rebuilds the overall metabolism of the body, can provide blessed relief and bring about eventual full recovery.

Remember These Important Points from This Chapter

1. There are different types of arthritis. The most common ones are rheumatoid arthritis, osteoarthritis, and gouty arthritis. Symptoms should be heeded, and at the slightest indication, a drugless, natural, corrective regimen should be adopted.

2. Exercise, diet, and special baths help to eliminate clogged waste products from the joints and promote the restoration of health.
3. Drugs often trigger attacks of arthritis as well as other side effects.
4. Adopt a raw, natural, health-building food plan.
5. Exercise to limber up "waste-clogged" joints, and drain congested tissues.
6. Follow a well-regulated program of living to restore the body to normal functioning and to uproot the existing arthritis condition.

HOW TO RECOGNIZE AND COPE
WITH VARIOUS RELATED TYPES OF
ARTHRITIS AND RHEUMATISM

The earlier you are able to recognize the various related forms of arthritis and rheumatism and the sooner you adopt the care that I am outlining in this book, the sooner can you prevent them from making deeper inroads in your body. Not all of these disorders begin alike or develop in the same way. Many are deceptively mild and slow-creeping and we only begin to become aware of their serious nature after they have reached a more advanced stage. This is why it is to your benefit to recognize them during the early stages so that you can nip them in the bud.

Ankylosing Spondylitis. A form of rheumatoid arthritis that can ultimately become extremely disabling is ankylosing spondylitis. This form of arthritis usually starts in the lower part of the back, but then gradually continues to creep up, and in many cases ultimately affects the entire spine. In time, the bones "freeze" or fuse together, producing the condition variously called stiff back, poker back, bamboo spine, Marie-Strumpell's Spine or Van Bechterow's disease. This type of arthritis seldom develops in "older folks." It affects mostly the young, lanky type of male, and strain or injury plus unhealthy living habits may get it started.

How to Recognize Early Symptoms. The disorder usually begins with extreme pains and interference in the movement of the sacroiliac joints, the joints of the lower part of the back. Severe pains and loss of movement are the initial warning signs. It causes a gradual destruction, narrowing, and eventual calcification of the sacroiliac joints. In many cases the calcification keeps climbing upward, and in the more severe cases ultimately causes complete ossification of the entire spine.

Frequently, the normal curve in the spine is lost, giving the so-called "poker spine" appearance. In some cases the upper part of the back becomes curved backward causing the so-called "hump." This in turn causes the neck to extend forward with the chin reaching downward. In some cases, the head becomes bowed down until the chin rests completely on the chest. In these cases it seems as if the chin has been cemented down in this position since it can no longer be lifted up.

In some of the more severe cases the ribs become attached to the spine and become completely locked. This interferes with breathing. Although ankylosing spondylitis attacks the spine, beginning with the sacroiliac joints and then gradually climbing upward, the knees and shoulders too may become affected. This only bears out my plea that early symptoms should be recognized and cared for to halt the progress of this type of arthritis which ultimately may cripple the entire body.

DANNY'S REMARKABLE RECOVERY

A most vivid example of what can be accomplished in these cases when taken in hand early enough came to my attention recently. I am referring to the case of 28-year-old Danny R.

At the age of 11, Danny began to feel severe pains in his legs and pelvic joints. Gradually the pains continued to travel upward and in time his whole spine including his neck became rigid and stiff. For seven years Danny was treated for t.b. (tuberculosis) of the joints, and as time went on his pains and stiffness only continued to increase.

Then Danny came under the care of an orthopedic physician who after extensive tests concluded that Danny was not suffering from t.b. of the joints but from an infectious form of rheumatoid arthritis known as ankylosing spondylitis or Van Bechterow's disease, the type of rheumatoid arthritis that I am now discussing. In treating Danny, the orthopedic physician prescribed cortisone, and while this at first provided great relief from pain, the crippling and stiffening continued to grow worse. His whole spine and neck grew increasingly more stiff and rigid and in time his spine, his legs, his shoulders, and his neck became completely deformed.

Then he met one of those natural health enthusiasts who explained to him what natural healing methods could do for him, and Danny looking for a way out, for any ray of hope, decided to try it.

Danny started with a 35-day total fast program. For 35 days Danny took nothing but three glasses of water three times a day.

This was the beginning of his salvation. When I asked Danny whether he had any qualms in undertaking this long fast, he made light of it and mentioned that the scriptures explain that in ancient times many followed such fasting regimens. Danny had a religious background and this apparently made it easy for him to adopt this program. Following his total fast, Danny started with a completely healthful vegetarian diet and for the last six years has been adhering to this diet. Here too, his religious training seemed to have a strong bearing on him, for he mentioned that the Essenes, a religious sect of olden times, followed an abstemious and vegetarian way of life.

He also commenced doing various exercises, later he became interested in yoga, started regular hikes, and as his joints became more flexible and free he sought further help by visiting a nature cure health resort.

Today, while Danny is still walking with a cane and has a certain amount of stiffness, his hips, his spine, his neck, and his legs have loosened up sufficiently to enable him to take long walks, to do any exercises he desires, to climb mountains without any difficulty, to bathe and swim freely. He has been able to accept a full-time job with an advertising firm and both he and his friends are amazed at what this type of care has done for him.

Danny's case only illustrates that these cases need not be

written off as hopeless, that even in the most difficult cases, a well-planned health-building program followed consistently can often provide most dramatic help.

Could Danny Conquer His Affliction Completely?

This was a question that his friend asked me. Nobody can tell with any degree of certainty whether Danny will make any further progress, but it is well to bear in mind that the body has a tremendous capacity for adjustment when we persist with the right kind of care. Danny still has some stiffness and rigidity left in his hip and in some parts of his spine. He still walks with a cane. But if he perseveres with his health-building program, I feel confident that more improvement is still possible. Nevertheless, what he has accomplished in the four years since he adopted this program borders almost on the miraculous.

A word of warning is in order in connection with Danny's experience. A prolonged fast is not essential to bring about the needed detoxification in these cases. Repeated short fasts or restricted dietary programs for detoxification purposes and a complete health-building program of living followed consistently will often serve the same purpose and provide the same results. A prolonged fast is best carried out under adequate supervision, and when this is not available, a less intensive program may be more advisable.

THE "PERMANENTLY RIGID SPINE" OF RUSSEL D. AND HOW HE WAS HELPED

Danny was fortunate in finding his way to natural healing before the vertebrae in his spine had completely grown together, since once this happens no amount of care can loosen them up again, and flexibility and freedom of motion is lost forever. This does not mean, however, that those in whom parts of the spine have already become completely ossified or fused should not try to obtain whatever help may still be possible.

Russel D.'s spinal arthritis started when he was 21 years old after an accident which injured the lower part of his spine. He came to see me seeking help when he was 50. At that time his whole spine up to his neck had already become completely ossified. The neck was the only part of his spine that had not as yet grown together, but it gave him a great deal of pain and he came to me in the hope that I would be able to provide relief and prevent the vertebrae in his neck from becoming permanently stiff and rigid.

His wife who has been under my care for an entirely unrelated condition and obtained excellent results was instrumental in getting him to consult me. Discussing his condition, she told me that Russel would awaken during the middle of the night and cry out with pain because his neck was tightening up, causing him untold misery.

My first instructions were that he adopt a more healthful diet plan. Russel was told to eat fresh fruits and vegetables, cottage cheese, baked potatoes, small amounts of lean meat or fish. All refined and processed foods were excluded. He was NOT to eat any sweets, cookies, cakes, pastries, ice cream, any fat or highly concentrated fat foods, or highly seasoned foods. These foods only led to the accumulation of toxic wastes in his system and added to his difficulties.

Russel was to do regular exercises. Two beneficial exercises that protected his stiffening neck from becoming completely ossified were as follows:

1. Stretching his neck as far as it would go by bending it first to one shoulder, then to the other shoulder.
2. Rotating his neck as far as it would go, first to one side, then to the other side.

He was to take regular sunbaths, weather permitting. The sun was to be directly "beamed" upon the back of his neck and the upper part of his back. The crown of his head was to covered. Nightly, he was to take hot epsom salt baths. Other exercises were also prescribed and he followed them faithfully.

The feeling of rigidity in the back of his neck gradually "melted" away. His neck regained complete flexibility and became completely free of pain.

Some Limitations to Recovery. In this type of arthritis we are often limited by the complete damage that has already set in. Where the spine has become completely fused, motion can no longer be restored. The most we can strive for in such cases is improvement in general health and keeping the joints that have not yet become completely fused from growing together.

How to Reverse Arthritis Following an Injury. Accidents will happen! Often, when the joints are injured and left weakened, arthritis may strike! This is because the weakened joint becomes a "point of least resistance" and then arthritis can easily develop. This explains why arthritis strikes many otherwise seemingly healthy folks after they have been in an accident.

To help prevent arthritis from rearing its ugly head, the use of the hot epsom salt baths, natural foods, one day per week fasting (with the juice of one-half lemon in boiled water sipped slowly at intervals throughout the day), and other sensible health care applied after the accident helps to rebuild and strengthen the injured joints and protects them against the onset of arthritis.

My plea to those who are unfortunate enough to become injured and later develop arthritis is this: Please do not seek momentary relief or "instant" relief through habitual drug taking. In doing this you are only deluding yourself. Pain-relieving drugs can blind you to the fact that you are developing arthritis, but they do not get you well! I urge those who have had an injury, to follow a healthful program until the effects of the injury have been completely obliterated. This means adhering to a natural dietary program and also the adoption of all the other health-building habits outlined in this volume. And if you are wise, you will continue to follow this healthful living program even after the obvious effects of the injury have been completely overcome, so that you make sure to continue to stay well.

Still's Disease: Arthritis in the Young. Another type of rheumatoid arthritis, a type affecting the young is Still's Disease.

Janet's Story. Janet is a living example of what can often be accomplished in this type of arthritis when the right care is provided. When Janet was brought to me about three years ago she was in really bad condition. Janet was then ten years old. And what a frightening sight she was when she was first carried into my office. Her back, her hips and her legs were stiffened and rigid, and while her knees and ankles were thickened, enlarged, and immovable, the muscles in her legs were shriveled up and completely wasted. Her hips, her back, and her legs, were also full of pain and taking any steps was entirely out of the question. Her fingers, wrists, and shoulders too were badly deformed. Her feet and her toes were like icicles, showing how bad her circulation was. And how pale, wasted, and anemic-looking she was!

Janet Reborn. You should see how well Janet looks now. With the exception of the left ankle in which motion has not yet been completely regained, all her other joints are practically free from all crippling, and her pains have completely cleared up. She acts like any normal child; she can walk, play, and perform various tricks with her body like any other youngster without any sign of pain or discomfort. The stiffness and cripping that still exists (and there is very little of it in any of the other joints except the left ankle) is gradually clearing up, and I am hopeful that with time practically all her crippling will be a thing of the past.

No Magic in Janet's Recovery. As in all other cases that I am describing in these pages, there was no magic to Janet's recovery. I employed the same basic approach of detoxification and of rebuilding the overall health of her whole body. A carefully planned diet, the hot epsom salt baths, a regulated program of exercises, and the other simple care described in this book did the trick. It did not come easily; it took time, but Janet is surely on the road to a complete recovery.

How to Recognize and "Beat" Bursitis. The bursa is a thin-walled sac filled with a viscid fluid that protects the joint against friction. Repeated pinching or pressure in the bursa produces increasing injury. There may be an occasional ache or twinge of pain which may be advance warnings that something is happening in the joint that must be guarded against. The accumulation of toxic or irritating substances or excessive calcium deposits keep causing irritation, and serum exudes into the region in an effort to dissolve or carry off the irritants. This causes pressure and inflammation. As the condition worsens, there is an acute attack.

Bursitis (an acute inflammation in the bursa) can happen in almost any joint of the body but most often involves the shoulder joints.

Symptoms. The victim may be awakened in the middle of the night with severe shoulder pains. The inflammation may spread over the whole shoulder. Slight movement is excruciatingly painful; the pain often extends down into the arm and fingers. There is visible swelling and redness and skillful fingers can often discern the presence of calcium in the joint.

Tissues Must Be Repaired. Calcium deposits are not so much the cause as the result. Decayed or broken down tissue attracts calcium anywhere in the body. The purpose is to repair the tissues that have become damaged because they have been drenched with toxic waste products carried to the area by the fluids of the body and the blood.

Natural Diet for Self-Cleansing. Again we see that drugs must be shunned as they do little else but mask the acute attacks, leaving the joints greatly weakened. Ultimately a chronic bursitis with extensive deposits of calcium is the likely outcome. The natural diet I prescribe for sufferers from bursitis calls at first for one or two days of complete fast and abstention from solid food for two or three more days. Afterwards, raw and stewed fruit and raw and steamed vegetables are permitted.

Natural Home Remedies. Sleep and rest are wonderful home remedies. So is the use of the hot epsom salt baths, followed by moist local heat compresses. This helps ease the pain in the acutely inflamed joint. In some cases, cold compresses applied following the hot bath are well tolerated and provide more rapid relief of pain. I also prescribe at first complete immobilization or great limitation of motion of the affected joint, but as soon as possible start with gentle exercises.

Contrast Temperature Applications for Acute Bursitis Relief

Local applications of heat or alternate hot and cold contrast applications are of tremendous help. A sling provides complete rest to the shoulder joint. Mild stretching exercises as soon as the acute symptoms subside help prevent the development of a permanently locked shoulder joint, a condition often called "frozen shoulder."

A Helpful Exercise for Loosening Up Bursitis. This is an exercise I call the "climb the wall" exercise. Place your hand of the affected side against the wall and with the fingers keep climbing slowly upward as far as you can reach, and then climb slowly downward. Repeat this exercise eight or ten times. Repeat it two or three times a day, and always keep trying to "climb" a little higher. This helps to loosen up the stiff and rigid shoulder joint and prevents it from becoming completely locked or permanently stiff.

HOW SPENCER H. WAS RELIEVED OF BURSITIS WITHOUT DRUGS OR SURGERY

Spencer told me that he was awakened one night by throbbing, pulsating pains running up and down his right arm from shoulder to finger tips, from finger tips to shoulder. "It felt like a hundred hot knives and searing pitchforks jabbing into my flesh."

Spencer's wife had to shave and bathe him. He was as helpless as a babe and just as irritable. Every step he took sent pains shooting through his arm and shoulder.

Spencer was placed on the program outlined above and within a few days obtained almost miraculous relief. He was then instructed to start with the "climb the wall" exercises. Another few days and his acute bursitis had faded away completely and he was able to resume all his normal activities. All he had to do was to keep on living the healthful way to avoid a recurrence of the condition.

Slipped or Herniated Discs. The articular discs between the spinal vertebrae are composed of semi-soft cartilaginous tissue. They cushion the joints, provide flexibility of movement, and protect the joints against friction and injury. They act in the nature of shock absorbers. The discs in the lower part of the back are particularly prone to strain or injury. This often causes a great deal of pain and suffering. Calcium often accumulates in these joints and intensifies the suffering.

*Agonizing Pains Similar to Other Severe Forms of
Back Arthritis*

Let me say at this point that many cases diagnosed as disc disorders do not always show true disc damage. Other forms of arthritis can cause similar severe pains and suffering. Calcium deposits settling in and around the joint areas can create agonizing pains even though *no* true disc injury exists. Under all circumstances, the whole body, not just the specific joint, requires care.

Program for Herniated Disc Relief. A patient with a "disc" problem was Paula P. This patient suffered for 18 years from this difficult disorder. A leading orthopedic surgeon insisted that she needed surgery to bring about cervical fusion if she was ever to be helped. Failure to submit to surgery would ultimately land her in a wheelchair and she would be crippled for life, he said. She refused surgery, but when coming to me after 18 years of care with this doctor, her pains were more agonizing than ever, and she consistently had to depend on drugs for relief. The attacks of pain recurred when the effects of the drugs wore off. She also suffered from extreme fatigue and digestive difficulties. I put Paula P. on this overall body health program:

1. *Diet.* Because of her digestive difficulties, I placed her at first on a soft, bland diet. (I describe this diet in a subsequent chapter.) Then as her stomach symptoms cleared up, I added some fresh fruits and small amounts of finely grated raw vegetables. Later, after her digestive difficulties had been completely overcome, she was able to adopt the complete health diet program which included the use of all raw vegetables and raw fruits, and she found it most gratifying.

2. *Rest.* I insisted that she retire at a reasonable hour and that she get an abundance of rest and sleep. She was to take a nap or a rest period for at least one hour after her noon meal, and also arrange for rest periods at other times whenever possible.

3. *Local Applications.* Her most severe pains were in the neck and in the lower part of her back. To help loosen up the stiffness and relieve the acute pains in her neck, I had her resort to repeated

local heat applications. Her back too had to be kept comfortably warm and relaxed.

4. *Exercises.* To further loosen up the rigidity and tightness in her neck, I outlined a series of gentle neck-stretching exercises. She was to keep the neck warm, and every morning and night was to stretch and bend her neck gently as I describe in the chapter on exercises. To build up her weakened abdominal muscles and strengthen the lower part of her back, I also recommended first the simple leg raising exercises, and later the more advanced leg raising exercises.

5. *Alleviating Psychosomatic Disturbances.* Mrs. P. possesses a fine, sensitive nature. To help her get well I had to make sure that she learned how to relax and how to develop proper emotional control. Patience, tolerance and understanding are valuable traits that must be developed since they contribute much to the enrichment of life. The highly sensitive person often becomes overwhelmed by the many problems that arise in daily life and has to develop a proper perspective so that she can take them in her stride.

Paula adhered closely to my diet instructions and followed the restoration program that I outlined for her in its entirety. Gradually, her pains disappeared and now she is in excellent condition. Actually, nature did the healing.

Easing Low Back Pains. "Low back pain" is a sort of catch-all phrase. It covers many types of back disorders including lumbago, as well as various forms of rheumatism or arthritis. Low back pain or forms of lumbago, rheumatism, or arthritis, may be caused by falls, sprains or strains, also by improper posture or poor walking habits. Various internal disorders such as constipation or some other abdominal disorders or weaknesses also contribute to pains in the back as well as to the onset of back problems.

Nature's Warning. Low back pains may be a sign of early or advanced forms of arthritis. They may indicate the presence of disorders in the sacroiliac or lumbo-sacral joints. Often, these pains are caused by pressure on the sciatic nerve (the largest nerve in the body which runs down into the thighs and legs). It may also be due to a disc problem.

Restoration Program. To ease low back pain, follow the well-regulated program of sleep, rest, proper diet, warmth and moderate exercises described in this book.

Natural Methods Help Myositis. This form of muscular rheumatism is also known as fibrositis. Myositis or fibrositis and arthritis are often closely interrelated. Rheumatism affecting the muscles and connective tissues is known as myositis or fibrositis, while rheumatism affecting the joints is known as arthritis. The two are closely related. They are often found together. To conquer this type of rheumatism all we have to do is to follow the plan of care that I adopted in Mary D.'s case.

MARY D. AND HER SELF-HEALING PROGRAM FOR MYOSITIS

When Mary D. walked into my office, she was on the verge of tears. She complained of excruciating pains in her shoulders, radiating into her chest and down to her wrists. She had difficulty in catching her breath. The pains around her heart were so bad that at times she thought she was having a heart attack.

I diagnosed her condition as myositis, a form of muscular rheumatism. This was not the first time that Mary had come to my office. Several years before, she had suffered repeated gallbladder attacks, shown signs of poor liver function and complained of many arthritis symptoms. She had also suffered from sinus trouble and various other catarrhal disorders.

Natural food and a healthful living program helped her then, but with time she became careless again and drifted back to some of her former unhealthy living habits. The results? Renewed rheumatic and arthritic manifestations.

I told Mary to stop taking liberties with herself and to resume her former healthful living program. Here is what I told her to do:

1. She was to start with a two-day juice diet with apple juice as the only food.

COPING WITH RELATED TYPES OF ARTHRITIS AND RHEUMATISM   81

2. On the third day, she was allowed to eat any fresh fruit whenever hungry. In the evening she was allowed to have a meal of finely grated raw vegetables, a small portion of lean fish or chicken, or baked potato (without seasoning or butter added to it) and for dessert (optional) a baked apple with no sweetening.

3. Nightly, a hot epsom salt bath before retiring.

4. Daily, the deep breathing exercises as described before.

5. Rest. No fatigue. Ample rest and relaxation.

6. Her feet had to be kept warm to establish a more even blood circulation. After one month of this program, the muscular rheumatism faded into dim memory. When discharged she was in perfect health. It is my hope, as with so many patients who have entered my office as "hopeless" arthritics and left as healthy individuals, that Mary D. and the others who adopt this plan of care will continue with it even when away from my personal supervision. There is no compromising with nature when it comes to health.

Chapter Highlights in Identifying and Resorting to Self-Treatment in Various Other Types of Arthritis and Rheumatism

1. Spondylitis, Still's Disease, bursitis, and other forms of arthritis or rheumatism should be recognized and uprooted in the early stages.

2. For a rigid neck, follow the exercises described.

3. Follow the self-help program to reverse arthritis caused by injury.

4. Young people's arthritis should be nipped in the bud with the natural healthful living plan described.

5. Adopt the natural home care and the various water applications recommended for relief of bursitis and low back pains.

6. Slipped or herniated disc problems also respond to this type of care.

5

HOW TO RESTORE THE FUNCTIONS
OF YOUR BODY'S ESSENTIAL PROCESSES
TO COMBAT ARTHRITIS

Arthritis does not stand alone! A successful program of arthritis care requires the building up of the circulation and the strengthening of the nervous system, as well as the rebuilding of the functions of all the major glands and organs of the body. In arthritis, as well as in most diseases, no single part of the body fails or falters alone. When one organ or part of the body begins to fail in its functioning, other organs or parts become affected. This creates an internal upset and the entire body begins to suffer in various degrees.

Total Rebuilding Is the Key to Real Help. To get well, arthritis sufferers must adopt a program of care that aims to eliminate the influences that have contributed to the development of all the existing deficiencies and disorders, and that promotes total rebuilding. The aim must be to build a clean and healthy bloodstream, to strengthen the nervous system, to promote the elimination of toxins, to restore normal body chemistry, to rebuild the functions of the glands of internal secretion, and to reestablish a state of equilibrium and balance.

Benefits of Internal Cleansing. To help your body rebuild itself to an arthritis-free level, your internal organs, the glands, and the various tissues and systems require self-cleansing or detoxification for the following reasons:

83

1. An accumulation of acid-ash residues that are not passed off through the normal eliminative channels tends to clog up the smooth working efficiency of the arterial and bone structures, leading to changes that ultimately foment arthritis.

2. The hollow body organs (nose, mouth, stomach, intestines, bronchial tubes, urinary tract) often fill up with a sludge called mucus. Mucus is discharged by the lining of these organs when they are irritated by certain toxic or foreign elements. This is the way the organs endeavor to protect themselves against further irritation by these various toxic elements. This toxic waste also contains sloughed-off cells and other debris that cling to the vital body organs and this interferes with their normal functioning. Joint stiffening, persistent aches of limbs, impaired functioning of arms and legs, often follows the accumulation of mucus and other toxic material in some of the vital organs of the body.

3. Internal toxemia sets up sites for arthritis. Toxic waste products accumulate in "pockets" of the skeletal structure such as the elbows, knees, spinal column, fingers, and the nape of the neck. Persistent irritation "chafes" and leads to spasms, contractions and congestion, and this ultimately leads to arthritis. Internal toxic refuse is often highly acid and creates a great deal of irritation. A self-cleansing program (such as follows) is aimed at removing these toxic wastes. It purifies the bloodstream and promotes drainage throughout the whole system.

Proper Drainage Improves Glandular Function. Internal toxins hinder the functions of the vital glands of the body and lead to arthritic changes. The functions of the pituitary gland, the adrenal glands, the thyroid gland, and the other glands of internal secretion are closely interrelated. These glands of internal secretion working in unison with the hypothalamus, the portion of the brain that controls the function of the abdominal organs, control the temperature of the body, sleep, the so-called "electrolyte balance," and overall body functioning. In arthritis just as in other diseases of metabolism, the functions of these vital glands have become greatly impaired. Through a self-cleansing program and adequate rebuilding care, we gradually reestablish normal glandular functioning and bring about a state of balance and health.

Cleanse Your Insides as You Cleanse Your Outsides. Acid-forming foods such as meats, fowl and white flour products should be restricted. An inside-cleansing program means increasing the intake of freshly squeezed fruit and vegetable juices. The valuable vitamins, minerals, enzymes and trace elements in the juices provide good, vital nourishment and help to promote internal cleansing.

How to Adopt a Thorough Internal Housecleaning Program

1. Start with a complete fast or a fruit juice diet, and follow it for at least two to three days or longer. When fasting, take nothing but plain water or water flavored with lemon juice whenever hungry or thirsty. Avoid fluoridated water. If the water in your community is fluoridated, use bottled spring water. When on a fruit juice diet, take one glass of juice about every two to three hours or whenever hungry. Sip your juice slowly or take it with a straw or glass tube. Avoid taking the water or the juice chilled and make sure that you sip it slowly.

If you find a fast or fruit juice diet too strenuous, start by eating only fresh fruits for three days or longer. Take one kind of fruit at a time, and take it whenever hungry or about every two to three hours.

In cases where the arthritis condition is accompanied by a digestive disorder which precludes the use of raw fruits or fruit juices, a soft bland diet as I describe it in the next chapter becomes necessary. Before you can hope to overcome your arthritis, your digestive difficulties must be overcome or brought under control, and in severe digestive disorders where foods or beverages containing roughage or causing too much acidity are irritating to the digestive organs, a carefully planned soft bland diet is at first essential.

2. Get your bowels well regulated. Follow the instructions presented in another chapter of this book, or take warm cleansing enemas when really needed or when uncomfortable.

3. Take your comfortably hot bath with one or two glasses of epsom salt before retiring. When getting out of the bath, do not dry your skin. Get into a robe without drying, retire immediately,

and make sure that you are well covered. If this makes you perspire, it is beneficial since it shows that your body, by way of the skin, is throwing off some of its accumulated internal toxic waste products.

4. Start your deep breathing exercises and make them a daily routine by following them regularly every morning and night. This increases the oxygen supply to the blood, to the internal organs, to all the tissues of the body, and helps to rid the body of many of its toxic residues.

5. Keep your feet warm to prevent chilling. This helps to overcome congestion and often alleviates pain.

6. Make sure to get enough sleep and rest. This strengthens the body and promotes more normal functioning of the internal organs, enabling them to do a more thorough job of throwing off accumulated waste products.

Rebuilding of the Nervous System Checks Arthritis

Fatigue, tension, wear and tear undermine the health of the nervous system and do much to impair the general health of the body and the mind. Stress often leads to symptoms resembling arthritis, and if continued, initiates the disease. The nervous system is delicate and reacts to stress with instant effect. To rebuild the nervous system, the first step is to change to a health-rebuilding diet and to get enough sleep and rest. Added to this we must also make sure that we develop a positive outlook on life. Eliminating negative and destructive thinking and developing an attitude of calmness and serenity, is a MUST!

Over-irritating Foods. Highly stimulating foods and beverages such as spiced meats, prepared and packaged foods, and bleached and chemically preserved foods, should be eliminated since they are destructive to the nervous system. Coffee, liquor, sweets, and sharp irritating condiments and spices are like toxic drugs. They impair the functioning of the nerves, they create a great deal of restlessness and often disturb sleep. This in turn depletes the nervous system even more. Return to a natural, wholesome diet. Restrict or eliminate completely the use of artificial foods and plan a way of life that strengthens and rebuilds your nervous system.

Nervous Tension. Too much of rush-rush-rush can make insomnia a lifelong habit and destroy you.

Your Stress-Easing Plan

1. Avoid the "Superman" urge. Do all that you can without straining yourself. Sometimes it *is* better to put off something that you have to do today for another day.

2. Noise-proof yourself. Insulate yourself from noises that get on your nerves. Get off to a quiet place by yourself and just relax. No radio, no television, no telephone. Also—no people! Give your nervous system a chance to regenerate its vital powers and regain its strength.

3. Enjoy recreation more than just on Sundays. Why not take more frequent weekend trips to the country? If possible, catch up on your work and take off an occasional afternoon for a trip to a quiet nearby country place, or just a jaunt in the woodsy area of your vicinity.

4. Stop pushing! Relax and let your tensions ease up. When the going gets rough, when problems become burdensome, just sit back, close your eyes, and stare at nothing with your eyes closed. Breathe deeply. When you return to your work, you'll feel refreshed and invigorated.

5. Try this stress-easing health tonic: use carrots, celery and apples, put them through a juicer, and sip the juice slowly. This is strengthening, invigorating and relaxing. Then lie down, make sure that your feet are warm, close your eyes, make your mind a blank, or if this is too difficult for you, start thinking of something that is pleasing and enjoyable—a new dress that you just bought and that you enjoy wearing, a contemplated trip and what you expect from it. Think of a recent happening that was gratifying, a story you read that gave you pleasure, dream or think of anything that is relaxing and pleasurable.

6. Here are some body stretching exercises that loosen up tight nerves and muscles. (*a*) Stand upright with arms stretched up-

ward over your head. Bend forward, trying to touch your toes with your fingertips, then straighten up and repeat. (b) Stand upright with legs spread far apart; then swing your body slowly to the right side, trying to touch right toes with left fingertips. Straighten up and then swing the body slowly to the left side, trying to touch left toes with right fingertips. Repeat two or three times and then gradually increase the number. (c) Stand upright with legs far apart. Reach with left hand to left side, trying to touch floor; then reach with right hand to right side. Repeat two or three times and then gradually increase the number.

Or if these exercises are at first too difficult for you, lie down on the floor or on a couch, close your eyes and do your deep breathing exercise. Breathe in deeply and slowly through one nostril five times, through the other nostril five times, and then through both nostrils five times. Follow with the milder leg-raising exercises, raising one leg three times, the other leg three times, and then both legs three times. Then relax and rest.

Digestion-Assimilation Aids to Overcome Arthritis

As stated before, arthritis does not stand alone; it is part of a whole syndrome of afflictions. Aside from those cases which develop solely as a result of trauma or local injury, the existing arthritis condition is a link in the chain of many bodily disorders. A poorly functioning digestive disorder is often one of them.

HOW DIGESTIVE IMPROVEMENT RELIEVED ELSIE'S ARTHRITIS

Elsie B. E.'s case history: 57-year-old Elsie B. E. has been suffering from arthritis for many years. It began with severe pains and aches in her collar bones but then the pains traveled to different parts of the body. She had pains in her fingers, pains and aches in her arms and legs, also pains and soreness in her breasts; but these pains were not really in her breasts, they were in her ribs. Elsie was head librarian in her home town, and the air conditioning where she worked only increased her pains. She suffered from cold hands and feet and became easily chilled. During the years, Elsie had been taking a great many drugs and at one time was told that traction would help. She tried it but it did not get her anywhere. As time went on her pains only became worse.

She also suffered from migraine headaches, and gave a history of ulcers which had cleared up. She was badly constipated and suffered from a spastic colon which caused a considerable amount of pain. She had been suffering from these pains for a great many years. Because of her spastic and irritable colon, Elsie had to avoid raw fruits and raw vegetables, and so I placed her at first on a soft bland diet; baked apple and baked ripe banana in the morning, baked potato and one to two steamed vegetables for lunch, a small portion of lean fish or chicken, and one to two steamed vegetables for dinner. Later when her spastic and irritable colon improved, I was able to add small amounts of finely grated raw vegetables and some of the bland raw fruits such as grated sweet apple, cantaloupe and papaya. Still later, other wholesome, health-building foods were added, and in time she had no difficulty in digesting all the raw vegetables and fruits that she wanted to eat.

I also advised much sleep and rest. She had to make sure not to become overtired. Mild physical exercises helped to rebuild the circulation and to strengthen her body. The hot epsom salt baths were relaxing and promoted the elimination of toxins through the skin. It did not take long before Elsie began to feel better. The soft bland diet relieved her digestive pains and discomforts, and as soon as these pains were relieved, other pains and aches began to lessen and finally cleared up completely. Now one year later, there is not a sign of her digestive upsets, her migraine headaches have entirely cleared up, her constipation is a thing of the past, and there are no longer any arthritis pains.

How to Use Your Lungs to Clean Out Your Insides

Each breath you take draws vital, life-giving oxygen into your lungs. This oxygen is taken up by the blood and then distributed to the body cells and tissues. Another vital function of the lungs is to expel the poisons that the blood brings back to the lungs from all parts of the body.

Clean, fresh air is vital to the maintenance and rebuilding of health. Those who live in large cities should arrange to take periodic vacations in the country. Deep breathing sends a flow of fresh oxygen to all the tissues of your body. It also "bathes" the bone marrow and helps to build a richer and healthier bloodstream.

A Highly Effective Deep-Breathing Exercise Program

1. Lie flat on your back with arms stretched out at your sides, palms downward. Keep mouth closed and inhale deeply and slowly through both nostrils, then exhale slowly, also through the nostrils. Relax and repeat.

2. Keep mouth closed and while keeping the left nostril closed with your thumb, inhale through the right nostril. Then while keeping the right nostril closed exhale through the left nostril.

3. Repeat the same exercise through the left nostril, inhaling through the left nostril and exhaling through the right nostril. These deep breathing exercises are highly relaxing and invigorating.

Kidney Health and Arthritis. Low back pains or a stiff lower back is often regarded as one of the many arthritis afflictions. Many of these pains can be traced to the kidneys. Here, the body's filter plant is at work. Daily, some 150 quarts of fluid pass through the kidneys, but only a small part of it is being eliminated by way of the urine, the rest is being reabsorbed. Each kidney is made up of a million or so tiny filters that strain waste products out of the blood, dissolve them in the fluid and then excrete them in the urine. The blood enters one end of each of these tiny tubules and is then propelled onward to the other and smaller end. This creates an effective filtering system. If this filtering system becomes faulty or breaks down, toxins accumulate in the tissues of the body, and ill health is an inevitable outcome.

How to Clean Your Kidneys

First, stop eating so that the kidneys can catch up with their backlog. Take water mildly flavored with lemon juice whenever desired, but nothing else. After two or three days of this program, start eating by taking fresh fruits only for one or two days. Take only one kind of fruit at a time whenever hungry or about every two or three hours. Then follow with a diet of fresh fruits all day and an evening meal of a large raw vegetable salad, a baked potato or small portion of your favorite protein, such as the soft cheeses, lean fish or fowl, or any lean meat, and one steamed vegetable. Take your hot epsom salt baths daily, and without drying, slip into a robe and get to bed. If this induces perspiration, fine! This only helps to throw off the poisons by way of the skin and lessens the burden on the kidneys. Also get enough sleep and keep your feet warm.

The kidneys should be kept healthy by being fed natural foods and they should be provided with other health-building care. Avoid salt, pepper, alcohol and artificial flavorings. These substances are excreted through the kidneys and have a harsh action on the tissues. They tend to poison the delicate filters and cells and impair their functions. Take fresh fruit and vegetable juices as part of your "kidney washing" program.

Why We Insist That Drugs Be Eliminated. Very simple. We do not wish to mask the disease. We have to uproot it, not mask it. Drugs hide from us the fact that we are sick and only mislead us by making us think that we are getting well. Furthermore, toxic drugs and chemicals further undermine the health of the body. Toxic drugs and chemicals have to be neutralized by the liver and have to be eliminated through the kidneys or the other organs of elimination. This only throws an added burden on the vital organs of the body. A drug-free plan brings arthritis to the surface. We then can see how sick we really are and understand the necessity of doing everything possible to uproot it.

Your Skin: The External Strainer

Your skin is a strainer. Through the millions of pores, accumulated sludge and debris is being excreted. Keep your skin cleansed by dry or moist friction rubs and comfortable hot baths.

And then follow the internal detoxification plan outlined above.

Use epsom salt, sea salt, or pine needle extracts for the bath for improved skin function. Many patients who come to me suffering from arthritis have an unhealthy skin, covered with sores, blotches, and various sorts of blemishes. With these baths and a change in their eating habits, toxic wastes are removed, blemishes clear up, and the function of the skin, the "strainer" of the body, is rebuilt. The pores become cleansed and unclogged, and internal poisons are released and thrown off. This helps to restore the body's equilibrium and facilitates the eventual restoration of the health of the arthritis sufferer. Whenever you wish to take a soap bath, use only a neutral soap free from sharp, irritating chemicals. These soaps are usually available in special dietary and health shops.

How the Colon Aids in the Elimination of Toxins. So much of internal cleansing depends upon the functioning of the colon, the lower portion of the gastrointestinal tract. The work of the stomach and the small intestine is to digest the foods we eat, while the large intestine (or colon) expels those portions of the food that have not been fully digested or that are indigestible. Failure of the colon to function efficiently leads to the retention of waste, causes a great deal of fermentation and putrefaction, and sets up a series of reactions that may contribute to the development of disorders that are related to arthritis, and eventually arthritis.

How to Improve Colon Efficiency. When people are constipated for years, they often consider their condition hopeless. But this is not the case. Just give up the clogging, putrefying, highly concentrated foods. Then use the raw vegetables and fresh fruits. They provide strengthening and rebuilding foods and help to reestablish normal bowel functioning. Follow your exercises regularly and get into the habit of trying to move your bowels naturally morning, noon and night. Before very long you will see beneficial results.

How Your Glands Can Ease Arthritis. The various glands of the body work together and pour out natural hormones. One substance produced by the adrenal glands is *cortisone*. Arthritis sufferers will recognize this as a chemical drug used in the treatment of arthritis. But nature has seen fit to supply us with cortisone the natural way by means of the workings of the various internal bodily glands.

How to Strengthen Your Glands to Produce Natural Cortisone

But when your glands cannot manufacture this substance, you do not help yourself when you try to get it artificially in the form of a medicine. Your own internal glands must be strengthened and rebuilt so that they can secrete this as well as other needed hormones. To strengthen and rebuild your glands, get enough sleep. Stop consuming stimulating beverages and foods. Discard all harmful influences that whip up the glands and get them overtired. Learn how to relax. The glands, like any of the other organs and tissues of the body, need kindness and good care to strengthen and rebuild them, and only when you adopt this well-regulated plan of care and follow it consistently will you succeed in rebuilding them. They will begin to function normally and this will restore balance and equilibrium throughout the body.

Restore Your Body Health. When normal body functioning is reestablished, renewed health is inevitable. When the entire body is rebuilt, all the organs and tissues of the body begin to function normally. Only by adopting the way of living that I am describing in these pages can you make sure of rebuilding the health of the whole body. *This is the only way arthritis sufferers can regain their health and overcome the disease.*

In this chapter I am trying to make clear what the arthritis sufferer must do to help restore better functioning and bring about a return to health. However, cases vary, and experience is often of great help in determining the modifications that may have to be made in each individual case. This is why I suggest that whenever possible you place yourself under the care of a doctor or practitioner who specializes in this type of care, the type of care that is based on sound biological principles and that helps to rebuild and regenerate total health.

Where this type of help is unavailable or impractical, you must still realize that only by adopting this natural, body-cleansing and body-building program can you attain the help you need. You must then carefully evaluate your own needs and then adopt the program to your own basic requirements. You must discontinue all body and health destroying drugs, and adopt a complete body and health building regimen. Do it intelligently and adhere to it faithfully and consistently. Get helpful advice if possible, but if this is not within your reach, you must still try to do what is best by following the program that I am outlining in these pages, since this is the only way you can obtain the help you need.

Highlights of This Chapter

1. Total body rebuilding is the key to arthritis relief.
2. Follow the internal cleansing plan by facilitating internal drainage.
3. Try the "blood-cleansing program" for a healthy bloodstream.
4. Relieve constipation with this natural, drug-free method.
5. Rebuild your nervous system and ease tension by following the special program described.
6. Arthritic relief is often based on proper assimilation of food as explained in the case history with its program.
7. Take a "lung purifying" bath to improve internal oxygenation.

HOW TO SELECT
HEALTH-BUILDING FOODS AND DEVELOP
WHOLESOME EATING HABITS

Nutrition plays a vital role in the uprooting of arthritis. A good nutritional program is essential because it helps to rebuild the overall health of the body. In arthritis, there is an upset in the delicate calcium-phosphorus balance and this is only one of many disturbances which proves the need for a wholesome health-building nutritional program.

How Correct Mineral Balance Relieves Arthritis. Too much or too little calcium deposited in and around the bones and joints tends to aggravate the arthritis condition. Excessive amounts of calcium deposited in and around the joints cause them to become calcified and thickened. Deficient calcium leads to osteoporosis or a weakening of the bones.

An imbalance of calcium and phosphorus usually exists in arthritis. This imbalance often is due to an impairment in the metabolism of the body, but is often also brought on by poor nutrition. This imbalance often contributes to the onset of arthritis, but also gives rise to many related disorders including anemia, poor circulation and an unhealthy nervous system, as well as an impairment in the functions of the endocrine system (the glands that secrete body hormones and regulate its functioning). This emphasizes again that arthritis is not a singular ailment, but one of a series of related internal derangements.

FOOD NOT A SPECIFIC REMEDY FOR ARTHRITIS

While there are no foods that can be considered as a specific remedy for arthritis, a well planned dietary program is essential if sufferers from this disease are to get well, since only a correct dietary plan can provide the minerals that are lacking in the body and that can help to rectify various existing weaknesses and disorders that have to be overcome if the disease is to be uprooted. This dietary program calls for the use of LIVE, VITAL, body and health building foods, and raw fruits and vegetables are among the foods that are most essential. It also calls for corrective eating habits.

HOW TO IMPROVE ASSIMILATION OF NUTRIENTS

While it is essential to eat wholesome natural foods, it is even more essential to strengthen and rebuild the functions of the digestive system so that the foods eaten can be properly digested and assimilated. Here is a guide that I have prepared for many of my patients to help them improve the digestion and assimilation of the LIVE, VITAL foods that I want them to eat:

1. Eat only when hungry. It is unhealthy to eat by the clock. Hunger is the guide to eating since this is the way the body tells us when its food needs have to be replenished. Appetite is a craving for food and not natural hunger. When you follow a healthy way of living, you will soon be able to distinguish between mere appetite and real hunger. You should eat only when you have a real need for food, not merely a craving for foods.

2. Eat slowly. Chew your food thoroughly. Take your time when chewing and enjoy every morsel of the food you eat. Chewing helps to improve digestion.

3. Eat until your natural hunger has been satisfied, and then stop! Do not overeat since this overburdens the digestive organs. It leads to excessive fermentation and much gas formation. Furthermore, certain undigested or indigestible food particles start

putrefying in the colon and toxic elements are created which are then absorbed into the system. Eventually, the mineral balance is upset and this leads to more intensified arthritis symptoms. Get up from the table feeling that you could still eat more, rather than eat until you feel stuffed. Learn to push your chair away from the table and get up before you feel full. Some may not find it too easy to do, but be assured that it will make you feel much healthier, and in the long run, much happier.

Live, Vital Foods Essential for Arthritis Correction. To restore the nutritional balance in the body, these LIVE, VITAL foods are a "must" in the arthritis sufferer's program for self-help:

1. Fresh fruits and raw vegetables. These foods are rich in essential minerals, vitamins and enzymes, as well as the very important trace elements. They supply appreciable amounts of protein which is valuable for the rebuilding of bones and tissues. They are the foundation stones for a restoration of health.

2. Importance of raw foods. To derive the most out of LIVE, VITAL foods, the arthritis sufferer should use an abundance of these foods in their uncooked form. The secret here is that many vitamins, minerals and enzymes, as well as some of the trace elements are destroyed or lost by cooking, and the body then fails to get many of these valuable substances. Raw foods are rich in these natural nutrients, and the arthritis sufferer needs them. Here are several points that those who suffer the tortures of arthritis and who wish to get well should remember:

a) Always make sure you eat at least one large raw vegetable salad a day.

b) When hungry between meals and the digestive system allows it, fresh, fully tree-ripened grapefruits taken between meals are best. They are valuable detoxifiers. One or two days a week on grapefruit exclusively is of great help.

c) Also periodic days on freshly extracted raw vegetable juices or fresh fruit juices provide valuable nutrients and help detoxify the body.

A Low Sugar Diet Restores Mineral Balance. Most sufferers from arthritis consume large amounts of carbohydrates, low in minerals and high in calories. Large amounts of carbohydrate foods—the refined flour and white sugar products, cookies, cakes, pastries, ice cream, pies—displace a comparable amount of foods that contain valuable nutrients, the nutrients that the arthritis sufferer really needs.

Sugar throws the calcium-phosphorus balance out of kilter. It causes a retention of calcium (thus clogging joints), while lowering the phosphorus. When this effect wears off, the reverse occurs, with the phosphorus level shooting up and the calcium level becoming depressed.

To restore the mineral balance in the body, all white-flour and white-sugar containing foods should be eliminated. Many of my patients recovered from their serious arthritis condition when they replaced their refined cereals, their white breads, and their cookies, cakes, pastries and ice cream with a diet of fresh fruits and vegetables. This change normalized their mineral balance.

Artificial Sweeteners Should Be Eliminated. All forms of synthetic sweeteners are taboo in the mineral improvement plan. These artificial sweeteners are coal tar derivatives, and are harmful to the body. The artificial sweeteners are chemicals. They have no food value and can be toxic. Avoid all foods and beverages that contain artificial sweeteners of any sort.

The Diet That Helped Mrs. A.

Mrs. A., 67 years old, was in bad shape when she was brought to me by her daughter. She was badly crippled and suffered unbearable pains in her knees, back, shoulders and chest. She could hardly walk, every step was agony. Her legs were heavy and swollen. Every move was torture. She also complained of terrible burning in her feet. She had high blood pressure and was greatly overweight.

What was her diet? Here is a sample of her daily fare before she started with our LIVE, VITAL FOOD Program. Do you see some of your own "taboo" foods in this diet?

Breakfast: French toast and salted butter or cereal with milk, and coffee. Sometimes crullers, a piece of cake or cookies.

Lunch: Eggs or bacon, bread and butter, coffee.

Dinner: Chops, or chicken, or fish, or some other type of meat, soup, a cooked vegetable, bread and butter, and coffee. Pie or cake with syrup.

Her New Diet Plan. I told Mrs. A. that she should begin her diet plan by keeping to an exclusive grapefruit diet for two whole days. During these two days, she was to eat nothing else. She was to take one grapefruit (without sugar or any sweetening) about every two or three hours or whenever hungry. After the first two days, Mrs. A. was put on a diet composed of fresh fruit only, to be taken until evening whenever hungry or about every two to three hours. Her evening meal was as follows:

1. A large raw vegetable salad of romaine lettuce or other available lettuce, escarole, chickory, grated carrots, grated beets, parsnips, turnips, green or red sweet pepper, cucumber, celery, watercress, or any available green or root vegetables. She did not have to eat all these vegetables at the same time; she could use any combination she desired and vary them. But the rule was that each and every main evening meal had to include a large RAW vegetable salad. For dressing, either lemon juice or a sweet and sour dressing made up of lemon juice and a small amount of honey was permissible.

2. A small portion of lean fish, fowl, or any LEAN meat, either broiled, boiled or baked. No fried foods of any sort.

3. One or two steamed vegetables. NO salt. NO butter. For flavoring, tomatoes, onion, garlic, dill, or any mild herb.

4. Dessert could be any fresh fruit or grapefruit but without any added sweetening.

This diet plan was followed by Mrs. A. for three weeks.

Second Diet Plan. By that time Mrs. A. had experienced much relief from pain and the second stage of the health restoration plan was put into use.

Breakfast: (1) A raw fresh salad, or seasonal berries. (2) A small serving of natural brown rice, buckwheat groats, millet, or any natural whole-grain cereal served with stewed fruit. (Examples are stewed peaches, apple sauce, baked apples or pears.) These foods should be eaten slowly and should be thoroughly masticated. You will find a wide variety of natural whole-grain cereals as well as millet, buckwheat groats, and natural brown rice at any good health food store. (3) A cup of alfalfa tea, mint tea, camomile tea, or sassafras tea, slightly sweetened with natural honey. Or a glass of raw skimmed milk. NO sugar to be added to the stewed fruit or to be used with any of the beverages. The milk was to be sipped *slowly* or taken with a spoon.

Lunch: (1) A large raw vegetable salad. (2) One or two steamed vegetables, or corn on the cob and one steamed vegetable, or baked potato or yam or sweet potato and one steamed vegetable, or whole wheat toast and one or two steamed vegetables. (3) For dessert if still hungry, a baked apple or stewed or soaked sun-dried unsulphured prunes; or any other unsulphured, natural stewed fruit.

Remember This: All fruits must be prepared without any sweetening. All vegetables must be free of salt or butter.

A "Health Lunch." A large fruit salad made up of fresh fruits and seasonal berries with a half-cup of cottage cheese, pot cheese, farmer cheese, or ricotta (Italian cottage cheese), or a portion of avocado. These are filled with body-enriching vitamins, minerals, enzymes, protein and needed calcium phosphorus.

Dinner: (1) A large raw vegetable salad. (2) A small portion of your favorite protein foods such as meat, fish, poultry, or any of the other protein foods mentioned later. (3) One or two steamed vegetables. (4) If still hungry, raw fruits or berries.

Wholesome Starch Food. The arthritis sufferer is often benefited when he occasionally skips his protein such as the meat, fish or cheese and replaces it with a wholesome starch food such as baked potatoes, yams, corn on the cob, or natural brown rice. This reduces the acidity in the body and helps to create the desired internal balance.

Why the Elimination of Caffeine Beverages Speeds Arthritis Relief

Coffee, tea, chocolate and cocoa, as well as the sharp spices and condiments, must be eliminated. Hot dogs, fried foods, pastries, cakes, cookies, all kinds of goodies, the cola drinks (which contain caffeine), the artificially sweetened drinks and alcoholic beverages must be excluded if the arthritis sufferer is to obtain the help he needs.

Caffeine, whether in coffee, tea, soft drinks, or any artificial food, stimulates the cerebral cortex, the thalamus, the vasomotor and respiratory centers, and influences the heat regulating mechanism in the brain. It hinders the cerebral (brain) blood flow. Many patients who are coffee addicts, suffer from insomnia, irritability, cardiac palpitation, tremor, convulsions, flushes, anorexia, dehydration, fever and overall discomfort.

It is also well to mention that caffeine-containing beverages increase uric acid, a substance that is known to influence arthritic conditions and plays a vital role in gouty arthritis.

The coffee break has become a regular routine in industry. Why not make it an apple or apple juice or some other delightful fruit juice break? This would be so much more enjoyable and could keep the person so much healthier and more efficient. And it would certainly be of help to those who are already troubled by the twinges of arthritis.

One patient told me of the fun and also of the benefits that she derived when instead of sipping coffee during the coffee break she sipped her "St. Patrick's Cocktail," the green vegetable cocktail that she brought along with her to be sipped when others had their coffee. She owned a vegetable juicer, and before going to work would extract her vegetable juice and bring it along in a thermos bottle, to be sipped during the coffee break. Ultimately several other workers in the shop adopted her idea.

How Coffee Affected Dr. J.'s Arthritis. Dr. J.'s experience with coffee only confirmed how harmful coffee can be to the arthritis sufferer. Dr. J., a 72-year-old orthodontist, seemed pretty frisky and young for his age, except for his hands which were crippled with arthritis. And you can well realize that in his work he needed his hands badly!

Dr. J. followed the detoxification program that I outlined for him and was greatly pleased with the results. He was able to carry on his work and the pains seemed to have cleared up entirely. That is, until he started "cheating" with his coffee, and then he found out how quickly coffee can reawaken pain and bring back the arthritis. "With the first cup of coffee I took, I felt the difference. Every time I take coffee, I invariably feel its effect on my arthritis," he said.

"My fingers are totally pain-free when I stick to my diet, but let me take a cup of coffee or even half a cup, and within half an hour, I have sensitivity in my finger joints."

An Artist's Gratitude. In my office hangs a portrait painted by Jane F. Jane's paintings were so well thought of that many of them were exhibited in leading museums. But Jane had become badly cripple with arthritis. She suffered badly with her back, had severe pains in her legs, and holding a brush in her hand was sheer agony. It took about eight to ten months or a year before Jane, following my health plan, regained her health and the use of her hands. Then, about a year later, in appreciation for what I did for her she painted the portrait that graces my office.

Benefits Described in This Chapter

1. A corrected mineral balance helps to overcome arthritis.
2. Assimilation of nutrients is essential for arthritis relief.
3. LIVE, VITAL FOODS supply *LIVE, VITAL nutrients* and help to bring the body back to health.
4. Omit table salt and speed up arthritis correction.
5. To maintain the mineral balance, avoid sugars, the refined and processed starches, and the sharp spices and condiments.
6. Eliminate caffeine-containing beverages for self-cleansing.

7

HEALTH-BUILDING
DIET PLANS THAT HELP THE
ARTHRITIS SUFFERER

Let us begin by considering the benefits of a mono-diet. A mono-diet calls for the eating of one particular food for a specified period of time or for the eating of one kind of food at a time. Stretching a point, this term is also applied to an exclusive all-vegetable or all-fruit fare, with abstention from other foods.

HOW A MONO-DIET HELPS IN ARTHRITIS

When fewer foods are eaten at one time, the burden on the digestive system is reduced and then the food can more readily be digested. As stated previously, what you eat is important *but what you assimilate determines the state of your health*. When you devote yourself to an all-fruit diet, you introduce a rich and *undiluted* treasure of vitamins and minerals to normalize your body chemistry. The presence of conflicting foods in your system often interferes with the digestion and assimilation of the foods you eat even when they are good foods. Eating too many kinds of food at any one meal also places an added burden on our digestion. On the other hand an all-vegetable diet which introduces tissue-saturating minerals that can perform their work without "competition" and dilution from other nutrients is supreme. It provides essential nutrients for body cell reconstruction and is of great help to better health.

The Vegetable Mono-Diet Program. Arthritis sufferers are in need of an abundance of vitamins, minerals, enzymes and valuable protein. Nature has put these valuable elements in balanced form in the green leafy vegetables; the protein in these foods is not in concentrated form and this is one of the secrets of vegetable mono-diet. It provides nutrients in their most balanced and most easily digestible form and without any excess of protein. Most people eat excessive amounts of protein under the mistaken assumption that a diet rich in protein builds better health. When the arthritis sufferer follows a vegetable mono-diet program for several days, he helps to establish a better chemical balance in the body, and this helps to rebuild his health.

How a Salt-Free Plan Helps in Arthritis. Salt is a burden on the kidneys. To conquer arthritis, all organs must be kept in a healthy condition, and this means that salt or sodium chloride or any food to which table salt has been added, should be avoided. Salt is eliminated from the system through the kidneys, and foods or beverages containing salt tend to damage or weaken these vital organs. Sooner or later the kidneys lose the power to discard salt from the body, and this often causes the accumulation of fluids. Use natural mild herbs or vegetable powders in cookery for cuisine flavor. They bring out the best in foods and soon eliminate the craving for salt. Natural mild herbs have no irritating effect on the kidneys or other organs of the body and make the foods most enjoyable.

Avoid These Salt-Containing Foods and Beverages

Avoid salted nuts, Nova Scotia salmon, salted or pickled herring, lox, other salted fish, salted cheeses, salted meats, salted canned foods, salted cereals, salted anything. They are poisons for you and you must not touch them. And don't be misled by the idea that because you perspire during the summer months, you have to take salt tablets. As long as you eat good, natural LIVE, VITAL foods, you get all the sodium your body needs in its natural form and you have no need to worry about not getting enough of it.

How a Salt-Free Diet Benefits Arthritis Sufferers. A salt-free diet releases the excess fluid that has been retained in the joints and tissues of the body and removes it from the system. This reduces swellings in the joints and lessens pressure and pain. It relieves the kidneys of the added burden of eliminating the salt taken into the system and gives them a chance to catch up with their work of detoxification. Salt irritates and tends to harden tissues.

Why You Watch Your Fluid Intake. Those who adopt this mono-diet health plan need not worry whether they are getting enough fluid into their system. We seldom find it necessary to drink water except sometimes when we are exposed over a long period of time to the hot rays of the sun, or when we are under a great strain. Our fresh fruits and luscious raw and steamed vegetables provide all the liquid we need to keep us well, and forcing ourselves to take more liquid than the body requires only places an added burden on it.

Make sure to stay away from drinking water except when you actually need it as when you are greatly thirsty or hot. And when you need water, use water that has not been fluoridated, or use spring or well water. Bottled spring water is easily obtainable in the larger communities. Fortunately spring water is inexpensive, and you should use it not only for drinking purposes when thirsty, but also for cooking, for your herb tea or your soup.

The Fruit and One Solid Meal Diet Plan. Those who find an exclusive fruit diet too difficult to follow, could have fruit all day until evening, using one kind of raw fruit every two or three hours or whenever hungry, and then eat a regular meal in the evening. This meal composed of a large raw vegetable salad, a small portion of lean fish or chicken or any lean meat, or baked or boiled in-the-jacket potatoes with one or two steamed vegetables (NO SALT OR BUTTER), is most nourishing. If still hungry, after a meal, a grapefruit or any other fresh fruit may be used for dessert with the protein meal, while a baked apple or any stewed fruit may be used with the potato meal. Again, NO sugar is to be added to any fruit, NO salt or butter to the vegetables. This

dietary plan will give you an excellent start and will lay the foundation for renewed health.

Incidentally, this is a most ideal diet for sufferers from arthritis
who also have to lose weight.

Advice for Those Who Cannot Handle Raw Vegetables. The
arthritis patient who suffers from various forms of digestive distress or certain other health problems that preclude the use of raw
vegetables or raw fruits will do well to adopt a soft, bland, nonfibrous diet and adhere to it until the associated health problems
that make the use of raw vegetables or raw fruits impossible or
inadvisable are cleared up or brought under control. Then raw
fruits and raw vegetables are gradually introduced. Here is an
example of such a diet:

Breakfast: (1) Baked apple or apple sauce with baked or broiled
ripe banana or plantain. (2) Cup of your favorite herb tea or
raw skimmed milk, sipped slowly or spoon-fed.

Lunch: (1) Baked or boiled-in-jacket potato or yam. (2) One
or two steamed vegetables from this group: carrots, parsnips,
turnips, squash, eggplant, okra. (3) Baked apple or any stewed
fruit.

Dinner: (1) Small portion of lean fish or chicken or any lean
meat. (2) Two steamed vegetables from lunch group. (3) Baked
apple or stewed fruit.

Baked apple or baked or broiled banana or plantain may also
be taken between meals and before retiring if hungry.

In cases of ulcer or other very severe stomach inflammation
small quantities of whole skimmed or diluted milk (diluted—½
milk and ½ water) taken between meals when necessary are also
beneficial and help relieve stomach distress. Freshly squeezed
grape juice diluted half-and-half with water is also soothing. In
some cases of ulcers of the stomach or severe stomach inflammation, a diet of raw skimmed milk for a limited period of time may
be most advisable. Small amounts of milk sipped slowly or taken
with a spoon or through a straw or glass tube when stomach pains
show up, is often very helpful. This is later followed by a bland,
nonfibrous diet, and raw foods are subsequently introduced after
sufficient healing and repair has taken place.

All foods must be eaten slowly. Take them in small quantities and chew well. It is better to eat more often than too much at any single meal. Milk when taken should be warm (never cold), but not boiled. No food or beverages should be taken too cold or too hot.

For those whose digestive problem is so severe that they cannot endure vegetables whole, vegetables and fruits pureed or grated fine before steaming to remove or break down fibers and coarse particles are recommended.

Benefits of Fasting with Emphasis on Arthritis Control

The body possesses stored-up energy much in excess of the energy needed for ordinary activities or regular bodily functioning. These stored-up reserves must not be squandered, and when they have been squandered they must be replenished. When we adopt a fast or limited diet program for a day or two or a few days at a time, we conserve bodily reserves and lessen the strain placed upon the digestive organs. This helps the body to rebuild the reserves that have already been wasted and is a step in the direction of renewed health. This also explains why the arthritis sufferer must not overtax his digestive system by eating too much food or the wrong kind of food, and why he must be careful not to combine foods improperly. The arthritis sufferer must rebuild his wasted energies, and when he abstains from food completely for a few days, or follows a more restricted dietary program, his digestive organs are given a chance to rest and this conserves and rebuilds bodily energy. Abstinence from food helps the body to dispose of toxins that have accumulated, and also provides rest to tired and overworked organs. This gradually strengthens and rebuilds the body.

The Value of Short Fasts. To detoxify the body, to rest the digestive organs and promote increased elimination of toxins by way of the kidneys, the intestines and the various other channels of elimination, try a short fast. At first, two or three or even more days. Then just one or two days a week.

How Often to Fast. Some keep their bodies in excellent condition with one or two fast days a week. If at all possible, make this a regular practice. However, if this is too difficult for you, resort to a fruit juice diet or a whole fruit diet one or two days a week as the next best substitute.

Your Beginning Fast. Prepare your digestive system for the fast by following at first a limited diet. Devote a day or two to liquids only. Take grapefruit juice or hot vegetable broth only (8 ozs.) about every two hours, or if this is too strenuous, adopt a fresh fruit diet for two or three days, taking one kind of raw fruit at a time about every two or three hours or whenever hungry. Or if you wish to do it at a slower pace, adopt a diet of fresh fruit only during the whole day, taking one kind of fresh fruit whenever hungry or about every two or three hours until evening, and then an evening meal composed of a large raw vegetable salad, baked potato or small amounts of your favorite protein food, and one steamed vegetable. Your system will then gradually become adjusted to controlled fasting.

What Controlled Fasting Can Do for the Arthritic

1. It hastens relief of pain.
2. It promotes more rapid elimination of toxins.
3. It prepares the body, so that it can undertake the task of total rebuilding, total rehabilitation.

How a Mono-Diet Helped Mrs. Olga E. I. This woman was stricken suddenly with unbelievably painful arthritis in both a shoulder and a knee. She had been suffering from recurring arthritis pains in the past, but this attack was the worst and most unbearable.

Mrs. I. was a business woman, dependent on going to business for her livelihood, and because of this attack was in danger of losing her position. In her own words, "I could neither pull myself up nor step high enough to get on a bus, and taxis became a financial burden. Previous attacks had all lasted well over a year, and I was desperately concerned."

This finally convinced Mrs. I. to adopt my program. I immediately put her on a raw fruit juice diet for two days, then on alternating special diet plans of raw solid fruits and raw solid vegetables. I prescribed exercise and a special diet with emphasis on natural foods. Also, hot steam baths (tolerably hot, that is) with epsom salts.

At first, the diet plan that I outlined for her seemed almost too difficult for her to adopt; she was over 60 and she thought that in urging her to follow a more limited dietary regimen I expected too much from her. Nonetheless she persisted, and while at first the pains grew worse, they then gradually began to lessen. "I could get out of bed in the morning without it taking fifteen minutes" she said, and then nothing could have persuaded her to stop with this care.

Some weeks later though, while continuing with her health program, she suffered what seemed to her like a terrific setback. Both legs erupted in a flaming rash. The pains increased to an excruciating degree and both legs looked as if they were completely on fire. But by that time she was fully convinced that the program she followed, with emphasis on fasting, a mono-diet, and other simple natural care, was the only correct approach, and although greatly concerned about this unexpected flare-up, she nevertheless agreed to abide by all my instructions.

It took several weeks before this acute flare-up and the nagging pains that accompanied it, subsided. By the end of four months, she was a completely new person. Not only had her acute attacks completely vanished, but also the nagging pains that she had known for years were gone.

Chapter Summary

1. Raw, uncooked foods on special diet plans exert an internal cleansing action; they help eliminate toxic residues.
2. A salt-free diet helps in arthritis.
3. There are important benefits from an all-day fruit and one solid meal diet.
4. Advice is given for those who cannot handle raw fruits and raw vegetables.
5. Controlled fasting gives internal organs an opportunity to recuperate and regenerate.
6. Special eating plans that have helped countless thousands of other arthritis sufferers are described.

8

HOW WATER
CAN BE USED TO BENEFIT
ARTHRITIS SUFFERERS

Water, when used correctly, can be of tremendous help to sufferers from arthritis. When used correctly water can be soothing, relaxing, warming, cooling, refreshing, pain-relieving. Just water, plain water, but when used right, it can do wonders for sufferers from this difficult and crippling disease. It can dispel pain, soothe the nervous system, promote the drainage of stagnant material, and be of great help in the rebuilding of the health of sufferers from arthritis.

HOW WATER APPLICATIONS HELPED MR. F.

This man suffered from a generalized arthritis but his knees were especially bad. His right knee would often swell up to more than twice its normal size. The pain was unbearable. The accumulated fluid was drained surgically and this gave him relief, but before long the fluid would accumulate again.

Cortisone and Aspirin Ineffective

Mr. F. took cortisone for close to two years; when he came to me he was taking twelve aspirins a day. Although at first doctors diagnosed his condition as chronic myositis and dermomyositis, the final diagnosis was that he was suffering from osteo- and rheumatoid arthritis. He was told that there was little chance that he would ever get well and that to obtain relief he would have to continue taking drugs all his life. At times he developed side reactions from the drugs and his condition grew steadily worse.

What Water Therapy Did for Him

First I placed Mr. F. on a careful dietary program. Then I instructed him to take hot epsom salt baths daily. Immediately following the hot bath he was to apply a moist, cool compress to the badly inflamed and swollen knee. The compress had to be well covered to make sure that it would get warm quickly and stay warm. I also took him off all drugs. Drugs provide temporary relief by suppressing the disease symptoms, but in time they make the disease only worse. Mr. F. continued these hydrotherapy applications right in his own home for five months. At the end of that time, his arthritis while not completely eliminated was nevertheless tremendously improved. The swelling in his knee had cleared up to the point where it was practically normal, and his pains were almost completely gone. While in the past, frequent tapping of the right knee was necessary to draw off the accumulated fluid and provide him with a certain amount of relief, during all the months that he was under my care this had become entirely unnecessary. The hot baths followed by the cold compresses, plus a careful dietary regimen helped to drain off the congested fluid from within, and the knee returned to its normal condition.

How Water Therapy Benefits the Sufferer from Arthritis. The hot bath promotes more rapid skin elimination and encourages increased kidney function. This helps to rid the body of the toxic wastes that have clogged up the internal mechanism of the body; it improves the circulation and provides great relief of pain.

Moist, Cold Compresses Necessary in Some Cases. While heat is usually most helpful in arthritis, in certain cases where the inflammation is of a severely acute nature, the application of moist, cool compresses or alternate hot and cold applications used in place of heat will often provide the desired help.

When moist, cool compresses are applied, they should be well covered so that the aching joint becomes warm, actually hot. It is this internal heat plus the dissolving effect of the water that helps relieve pain in these cases and provides the needed relief. When the moist, cool compress gets really warm, it can then be changed to a new one, and this too must be well covered so that it warms up or gets really hot again.

Here let me give you a word of warning. When I say a moist, cold compress, I mean a moist, cold compress, not an ice pack. A cold, moist compress helps to improve the circulation to the part to which it is applied and when well covered gets really warm, often actually hot, while an ice pack inhibits circulation, which is the *opposite* of what we need in these cases.

How a Hot Epsom Salt Bath Detoxifies the System. Comfortably hot baths, to which two glassfuls of epsom salt (or sea salt) are added, are most beneficial. These baths should at first be taken daily; but then may be reduced to one every second day. The baths are best taken before retiring since in most instances they relax the body and induce sound sleep. To maintain the bath at an even temperature, the hot water should be kept dripping into the tub while the bath is taken.

Following the hot bath, the arthritis sufferer should, *without drying*, immediately get into a robe and then retire. He should make certain to be well covered, and if this induces sweating, he should not let this worry him for this is only helpful.

The "secret" here is that in causing perspiration, toxins are being eliminated by way of the skin. These hot baths also induce more active kidney elimination.

Hot epsom salt baths can be used with great benefit in most cases of arthritis. They are usually relaxing and induce sound sleep. In some cases, however, they have an opposite effect. For some the baths may be too stimulating and then keep them wide awake. In these cases the hot baths should be taken in the morning or during the day, but they should always be followed by a period of rest, lasting from 30 to 60 minutes.

Stay in the bath for about 10 to 15 minutes, never more than

20 minutes. If this length of time is too wearing or makes you uncomfortable, reduce the time limit. Make the bath comfortably hot, and keep it comfortably hot while you are in it by letting the hot water drip in, but make sure that it does not get too hot if you are to get the most benefit from it.

While taking the hot bath, make certain that either a window or the door is kept slightly open to permit ventilation and prevent the air in the bathroom from becoming too stifling.

The Hot Mustard Foot Bath for Arthritis Relief. Where the arthritis sufferer finds it difficult to get in or out of a bath tub, hot mustard foot baths can be used in place of the hot tub bath. This too increases the circulation and provides great help. Fill a large bucket with hot water and add one or two tablespoons of dry mustard to the water. Mix the mustard thoroughly until it is completely dissolved. Soak your feet in this solution for about 15 to 20 minutes. While soaking your feet in the foot bath, keep adding hot water to keep it comfortably hot. Where 15 to 20 minutes proves too strenuous, reduce the time limit.

When finished, sponge off your feet with a damp, cool cloth. Do not dry, just sponge off and without drying get immediately into bed. Cover yourself comfortably and relax or take a nap.

Moist Hot Compresses for Local Arthritis Pain Relief. Take a piece of woolen or flannel material large enough to be folded two or three times. Use a Turkish towel if other material is unavailable. Fold it to proper size, dip it in the hot water, wring out the water but do not make it too dry, and then wrap it around the painful and inflamed joint. Cover it with a piece of oil silk or other plastic material so that the heat is retained. Then cover with another piece of woolen material or flannel, or with a Turkish towel. If necessary wrap a woolen blanket over it. Keep this on for about 45 minutes to one hour. Make sure that it is hot when it is applied and that it is well covered so that the heat is retained. Afterwards, remove the wet towel, sponge off the joint quickly with a moist, cool towel, and then cover it to keep it comfortably warm.

Alternate Hot and Cold Compresses for Great Benefit. This method helps promote drainage and rebuilds the circulation o.

the inflamed joint. When pains are acute and sharp and the joint is feverish and swollen, alternate hot and cold compresses promote the circulation and help drain off toxic waste products. It is best to begin with the hot compress first, keeping it on for 10 to 15 minutes, and then follow with a cold compress which is kept on until it gets thoroughly warm. Or take a hot epsom salt bath first, and immediately after the hot bath apply a moist, cool compress and keep it on for 45 to 60 minutes or until it gets very warm, actually hot. After removing the compress, sponge the part off quickly with a moist, cool cloth after you remove it, and cover well.

How to Apply a Cold Compress. Take a double layer of woolen material or flannel; dip in cold water, then wring it out but don't make it too dry. It should contain sufficient moisture to bring about a desirable reaction. Then apply it to the inflamed joint. Cover it well and leave it on until it gets very warm or even hot. When the compress gets hot quickly, it may be removed sooner and another moist, cool compress can again be applied.

Always finish with the cold compress; but make sure that the cold compress gets thoroughly warm before it is removed.

Keep remembering that if a cold compress is to benefit you, it must get thoroughly warm or even hot. This is why I stress that no ice packs but moist, cold compresses be used. An ice pack cools the part, but does not bring about an improvement in circulation, while a cool, moist compress, by getting thoroughly warm, does much to improve the circulation to the affected part and helps promote the drainage of congested matter. To obtain the greatest amount of benefit, these compresses must promote an increase in the circulation of the affected joint, not merely cool it. In cases where the patient's health is badly depleted, cool, moist compresses sometimes fail to warm up sufficiently to make them of value. In such cases, a hot water bottle or a heat lamp applied over the compress helps to get it warm and is often helpful.

Warm, Cleansing Enemas for Internal Cleansing Benefits. Use plain lukewarm water to which a small amount of table salt has been added. Add one teaspoon of table salt to one pint of water, two teaspoons to one quart of water, or one full tablespoon of salt to two quarts of water. Never use more than one quart of water at one time since too much water used at one time tends to distend the colon and often creates needless discomfort. In some cases, an enema made with only one pint of water may be adequate and more desirable, even though it may have to be repeated.

Benefits of a Warm Cleansing Enema. It promotes the elimination of stagnant accumulations from the colon, relieves flatulence, improves the abdominal circulation by removing obstructing wastes, and helps to break up congestion. It also reduces the strain on the heart as well as on the other internal organs of the body such as the liver, the gallbladder, the pancreas and the lungs.

Use Warm Cleansing Enemas with Care. Use warm cleansing enemas with care and only when they are actually needed. When used too often they tend to wash away the natural secretions, and cause needless irritation to the inner lining of the colon. They have to be used very cautiously in cases of spastic or sensitive colon and should be completely avoided in acute appendicitis or other acute intestinal inflammations such as ulcerative colitis, ileitis and diverticulitis. It is well to bear in mind that under certain conditions even such a simple measure as an enema has to be used with care and at times has to be completely avoided.

Enema Nonhabit Forming. As an aid to the problem of constipation, the use of the enema is advisable. It is nonhabit forming. Only stimulants or sedatives are addictive. Many people shy away from the enema, yet resort to laxatives or cathartics which are not only habit-forming but actually weaken the intestinal tract. The enema neither rebuilds nor strengthens the colon. It merely removes the accumulated residue and should be considered a temporary expedient until the necessary corrective measures have strengthened the colon and restored normal intestinal functioning.

Overcoming Pain the Natural Way

The arthritis sufferer wants to get well, but in the interim he also strives for relief of pain. This is where nature and natural treatments come in. Drugs or remedies that mask pain, in the long

un create only more disease and greater crippling. Natural healing is opposed to the use of drugs. On the other hand, the various
hydrotherapeutic (water) applications described in this chapter,
and the other simple natural measures presented in other parts
of this book, while not interfering with the body's innate efforts
to promote healing and repair, in time bring about relief of pain,
make the arthritis sufferer more comfortable, and help to bring
about the needed correction. What is even more essential, it helps
us to dispense with the use of drugs, which in the long run create
only a more chronic and intense form of arthritis, and, through
their dangerous side effects, often lead to other serious health
problems. We must always remember that suppression, while
sometimes providing temporary relief of pain, does not restore
the health of the patient.

When Cold Baths Should Be Avoided. Cold baths or cold applications intensify arthritis pains and as a rule should be avoided.
They cause too much of a shock to the system and lead to stagnation in the joints. A moist, cool compress may be used after a
hot compress or a hot epsom salt bath when necessary, and it may
be applied where hot baths or the application of heat causes more
intense pains, but as a general rule, heat in arthritis is best. Moist,
hot compresses or other forms of heat have a soothing and warming effect on the painful joints and often bring about meaningful
relief of pain and comfort. When using a cold compress, make
sure to have it well covered with a dry flannel or a Turkish towel,
since the compress has to get warm to be of any real value.

Local Hot Paraffin Baths Offer Relief of Pain. Various other
local applications of heat often provide relief to painful joints.
One of these applications is the hot paraffin bath. The hot paraffin
bath locally applied improves circulation, encourages the dissolu-
tion and reabsorption of stagnant material, and helps break up
congestion. It also has a soothing effect on the nerves of the inflamed joint. It often brings about a gradual relief of pain since
it improves the circulation in the joint and helps to carry off stagnant toxic material.

How to Make a Hot Paraffin Bath. Take three pounds of
paraffin and one pound of vaseline, and melt in a double boiler.
Be sure to keep the paraffin away from the open flame. Let it

cool until a thin white coating forms on top. Then dip your hand in the cooling paraffin and remove immediately. After the fine film of paraffin on your hand has become congealed, repeat the dipping until five coatings have been applied. While dipping do not move the fingers. The film of paraffin formed on your hand is like a thick glove. Keep the paraffin coating on your hand for 30 minutes, then peel it off like a glove. The paraffin can then be used again and again.

Apply the melted paraffin to joints that cannot be dipped into the solution by using an ordinary brush. Apply several layers and the beneficial effect will be the same.

Other Applications for Painful Neck or Any Painful Joint

1. Fill a bag or sock with heated sand or salt. Then wrap it around the neck and cover with woolen material or a Turkish towel. Keep it on for an hour or longer.

2. Use an electric pad at low heat. Cover the electric pad with a cloth or towel to protect the affected body part from getting burned.

3. An old-fashioned hot water bottle or a brick heated in an oven and then wrapped in some woolen material or a Turkish towel and applied to the neck or any other affected joint, is remarkably helpful.

4. Use flaxseed poultices, oatmeal poultices, or heated antiphlogistine (available at most pharmacies) and apply locally. Be careful not to apply antiphlogistine too hot since you can easily be burned.

5. Infrared ray lamp or any other heating lamp as well as a U-shaped baking lamp, holding 40 to 60 watt bulbs, can be used on the painful parts to provide relief. These lamps are sold in surgical supply outlets as well as specialty health stores.

How to Steam a Painful Arthritis Joint to Loosen Up Stiffness and Drain Off Toxins

Place a hot, moist compress over the painful joint. Cover with flannel, woolen material, or a Turkish towel, apply the heat lamp, infrared lamp or the U-shaped baking lamp over it for 30 to 45 minutes. You may use this steaming process twice daily or more often if necessary. This steams open the pores and helps to rid the affected part of accumulated waste substances. After removing the compress, sponge off quickly with a tepid or cool cloth and relax or take a nap.

Hydrotherapy Provides Lasting Benefits. Baths and other forms of water application when used in the right way help to rebuild the circulation, carry off toxic material, and start the body on its self-recuperative program.

These treatments encourage more normal functioning, the body gains in endurance and strength, and this ultimately leads to improved health.

Necessity of Moderation. Hydrotherapy provides more lasting benefits because it promotes better elimination by way of the skin. It also promotes elimination of toxins through the kidneys and in various other ways. But like any other method, these treatments should be used with moderation since when overdone, they could also have a depleting effect on the body. Furthermore, they do not correct the underlying causes of the disease. To obtain permanent results, a well-balanced program of living as outlined in this volume must be followed, since only when the chemistry of the body and the functioning of the whole body is restored to normal, can lasting results be obtained.

Benefits from Climatic Changes Are Minimal. Moving to a warm and dry climate often provides a certain amount of relief, but this does not offer real or permanent correction of the arthritis condition. Remember that no matter where you go you take your body with all its disorders and all its bad habits along with you. The only way you can get well is when you discard all unwholesome living habits and adopt a plan of living that restores normal functioning. A pleasant climate may temporarily make you feel better, but unless you recognize the need for a complete reformation in your mode of living, your desire to overcome your arthritis will prove to be just a hope.

Chapter Summary

1. Special compresses of moist wrappings improve the circulation to the joints and increase the elimination of poisonous wastes.

2. A hot epsom salt bath promotes the elimination of toxins through the skin and kidneys.

3. Mustard foot baths help relieve leg arthritis, and are also of great help to the patient who is unable to get into a hot bath.

4. Hot compresses soothe and relieve affected arthritis sites.

5. Alternate hot and cold compresses are often of great help.

6. Establish internal cleanliness with a warm cleansing enema when necessary.

7. Paraffin baths "pep" up blood flow to stiff and painful joints.

8. Use alternate self-help programs for relief of painful neck and other painful joints.

9. The effects of moving to a different climate are minimal.

10. To overcome arthritis, an overall health-rebuilding program must be planned.

EXERCISES AND HELPFUL MANIPULATIVE TECHNIQUES TO LOOSEN STIFFENED ARTHRITIC JOINTS

Many arthritis sufferers are discovering that deep body massage and a well-planned program of physical exercises, as well as various manipulative techniques can be of great help to them. When applied correctly these manual types of care improve circulation, loosen up rigid and stiffened joints, and do much to relieve pain and discomfort. Arthritis victims who complain of backaches, shoulder pains, and various other joint pains often obtain great relief from various manipulative treatments such as chiropractic, osteopathy, deep body massage and compression therapy. As an osteopathic, naturopathic and chiropractic physian, I have helped many arthritis sufferers towards their recovery by various body and joint manipulations as well as by the various manipulative techniques and self-applied exercises that I have encouraged my patients to adopt and carry out regularly in their own home.

How to Relieve a Rigid, Stiff and Painful Neck

Repeat the following movements regularly, five times each morning and night. Do them slowly. Stretch as far as you can in each direction. Performed regularly, these exercises loosen up stiff and rigid neck muscles and provide considerable relief of pain.

1. Sitting up, look straight ahead and relax. Then rotate your

head slowly, first to one side, then to the other side. Repeat five times.

2. Same position as No. 1. Bend head slowly, first to one side, then to the other side. Repeat five times.

3. Same position as before. Look straight ahead. Then thrust your head forward as far as it will reach. Return head to normal position and repeat five times.

4. Bend head downward to rest chin on chest. Then without lifting your head, push it backward. This is excellent for the upper part of the spine.

How to Relieve Severe Shoulder and Upper Back Pains

1. While in sitting or standing position place your hands on your shoulders. Then rotate shoulders five times forward, then five times backward.

2. Same position as before. Bend the upper part of your body, first to one side, then to the other side. Repeat five times.

How to Loosen Up Low Back and Hip Joints

1. Lie flat on your back. Place your hands at your sides and relax. Then without bending your knee, raise one leg up slowly as high as you can reach, and then bring it down slowly until you touch the floor. Pause, and repeat three times.

2. Repeat the same exercise with the other leg.

3. Repeat the same exercise with both legs. Begin by doing these exercises three times at first, then increase gradually until you are able to do them ten times. Bring your legs down slowly and pause between each movement.

Advanced Leg-Raising Movements

These exercises are to be added after those described above have been followed for some time and have loosened up the joints of the back sufficiently to enable you to include them without too much strain on your body.

1. Position as above, lying flat on your back. Raise one leg slowly as high as you can reach. Then swing it slowly over the

other leg, then bring it all the way back to the other side, then swing it to the center and lower slowly. Repeat three times.

2. Repeat the same exercise three times with the other leg and then with both legs.

Leg Resistive Exercises

Lie flat on your back. First bend your knees, then against resistance push them sideways, opposing the movement with your hands. Then bring them together again, also against resistance. Repeat five times.

Back Strengthening Exercises

1. Lie flat on your abdomen and slowly raise one leg backward as far back as you can reach, then lower it. Repeat 3 to 5 times. Repeat the same movement with the other leg. Then repeat the same movement with both legs.

2. Keeping the same position, raise one leg as far back as you can reach, then move it slowly outward, then bring it back and lower it slowly. Repeat 3 to 5 times. Repeat the same movement with the other leg.

Self-Manipulative Exercises for Stiff, Rigid, Painful Feet

In lying or sitting position:

1. Move both feet slowly up and down as far as you can reach. Repeat ten times.

2. Swing feet slowly from ankles, first inward, then outward. Repeat ten times.

Exercise for Greater Toe Flexibility

This is a "pencil grabbing" exercise, an exercise that brings greater flexibility to toes and feet, and helps in rebuilding the circulation in the feet. Use your toes as if you were trying to pick up a pencil or marbles, then release. Repeat ten times.

Exercises for the Wrists

1. Move hand slowly up and down, ten times.

2. Move hands slowly sideways, first in one direction, then in other direction, ten times.

Exercise for the Hands

1. Close fist slowly, then open up spreading fingers apart. Repeat five times and gradually increase to ten times.

Caution: Never force any movement. Extend each movement as far as possible, but do not force. In time the joints begin to loosen up and the range of motion increases.

The Value of Deep Breathing Exercises

The key to success in deep breathing exercises is in the intake of fresh, pure oxygen and in disposing of carbonic acid gas. Your body stores food, produces energy, maintains a stockpile of nutrients—*but it cannot store oxygen.* All the cells of the body need oxygen, and the joints of the arthritis sufferer are starved for it. The arthritis sufferer needs oxygen which is carried by the blood to the small hidden pocket sites where pain and crippling is often pronounced. Oxygen delivery is often deficient in these joints and this is where deep breathing and other exercises are of great benefit.

Your lungs should be thoroughly utilized to provide healthy, nourishing oxygen to all parts of your body. Deep breathing exercises—

a. enable the lungs to process more air with less effort.

b. strengthen the heart so that it can pump more blood with each stroke, reducing the number of "necessary" strokes. The heart of the well-conditioned arthritis sufferer on the road to recovery often beats 20 times per minute less than the non-conditioned arthritis victim. This saves the conditioned arthritis sufferer as many as 10,000 beats in one night's sleep—or up to 30,000 beats every day of his life! And just think how much energy your heart saves this way!

c. These deep breathing exercises help to increase the number and size of the blood vessels that transport blood to the body tissues.

d. They help improve muscle and blood-vessel tone and also help to reduce blood pressure.

e. When you walk, you help stimulate the flow of oxygen to all parts of the body in need of this inner "air bath."

HOW THESE EXERCISES HELP YOU FIGHT ARTHRITIS

As these exercises increase the size and number of blood vessels, new routes for the delivery of more oxygen develop. This is a vital factor in the health of the arthritis sufferer. When the heart is saturated with healthy blood vessels, the chance of cardiac failure is reduced. A healthy heart is also able to maintain a more efficient circulatory system which is of prime importance in arthritis. It not only helps the heart, but in helping the heart, the circulation to the joints is also strengthened and rebuilt.

Deep breathing exercises provide a deep sense of well-being. They develop better chest muscles, strengthen the abdominal muscles and are also highly invigorating. They start the day off just right.

During the day, when under tension, you can enjoy a greater sense of relaxation by getting away from your tasks and stretching out on your back, resting and relaxing completely and doing some deep breathing exercises.

REMEMBER: Deep breathing exercises are most effective when done slowly, rhythmically. If it is inconvenient to lie down, do them before an open window. But be sure that you inhale and exhale slowly, deeply, rhythmically.

Stretching Exercises. Stand up straight. Lock your hands behind your head, then slowly stretch them upward against resistance while rising slowly on your toes. Now stretch, stretch, s-t-r-e-t-c-h, S-T-R-E-T-C-H.

Rotating Exercises. Stand up straight, place hands on hips and rotate your body slowly, first to one side then to the other side. Rotate as far as possible. Repeat five times.

Posture-Building Exercises

Always maintain good posture: Arthritis sufferers often assume a slumping position which causes fatigue. This, in turn, leads to pain and ultimately stagnation, congestion, and a worsening of the arthritis. Try these posture building exercises and do them at least twice daily:

1. *In Standing Position:* Stand against a straight wall. Your feet together, place entire body including your head against the wall. Pull stomach in, tightening buttocks and press shoulder blades against the wall and slightly up. Then stretch tall, tall, tall. While stretching your body downward from the hips, let your head reach upward for the stars. Keep arms straight alongside the body and maintain this position to the count of 30. Then relax for one minute and repeat twice more.

2. Repeat the same exercise while lying on your back.

3. *In Sitting Position:* (For those who are unable to stand up) Repeat the same exercise in sitting position. Use a chair with hard seat and straight back. Touch the back of the chair with the back of your body. As above, pull stomach in, tighten your buttocks, and press shoulder blades against the back of the chair, and slightly up. Then stretch your head upward. Keep this position to the count of 30, then relax for one minute and repeat twice more.

How to Get the Most Out of Your Exercises

1. *Exercises Should Be Done Slowly and Rhythmically.* As an example, when doing your simpler leg raising exercises: Raise your leg up slowly, pause for a few seconds, then lower it slowly. Or when doing the more advanced leg raising exercises: Raise your leg up slowly, pause for a few seconds, then swing it slowly all the way over to one side. Pause again and then swing it over slowly to the other side. Another slight pause. Then bring it back to the center and lower it slowly. Pause again, and then repeat all over again.

2. *Exercises Should Be Carried through the Full Range of Motion.* Extend each movement as far as you can reach and you will find that gradually the joints will become more flexible and you will be able to do each exercise with greater freedom and ease. Pains too will lessen.

Exercises done regularly and consistently, help to loosen up and eliminate calcium deposits. Be careful not to overdo. Alternate the exercises with sufficient rest and sleep.

3. *Don't Let Pain Dissuade You from Doing Your Exercises.* Some pain is to be expected, since joints and muscles that have become stiff and rigid are being stirred up and reawakened. Adjust the exercises to your condition. Do the milder ones first and add the more strenuous ones as you get more limber and strong.

4. *Discontinue Exercises Temporarily When Pains Become Acute.* When acute pains set in discontinue the exercises temporarily, but get back to them as soon as the acute pains lessen. Never force your body to do the impossible. And be consistent. Do as much of the exercises as you can once or twice daily, and make sure that you fit them into your regular program of self-restoration and rebuilding.

5. *Do Your Exercises When Most Convenient.* For greatest benefit, make sure that when you start these movements your body is warm and relaxed.

Deep Compression Therapy: I pointed out before that certain manipulative techniques when applied correctly are often of great help in arthritis, and one of the techniques that I mentioned was compression therapy also known as zone therapy. This technique applied to certain pressure points in the feet helps to loosen up crystalline deposits and reflexly provide great benefit to the whole body of the arthritis sufferer. The crystalline deposits which accumulate in the joints cause pressure, irritation, and interference with freedom of movement. Gravity plus the special strains to which our feet are subjected often favor the accumulation of these concretions in the joints of our feet. This causes pressure on the delicate nerve endings in the feet and reflexly affects the health of the whole body. Firm, deep manipulation of the joints in the feet helps to loosen up and eliminate these concretions and this in turn helps the whole body.

The Benefits Derived from Manipulative Techniques Skilfully Applied to the Back

"*Go easy on my back!*" How often have I heard patients say this, and you cannot blame them since so much of their arthritis is located in the back, causing a great deal of agony and pain. This is why I advise that the utmost care be used in the application of chiropractic, osteopathy, or any of the other related types of mechanotherapy. These treatments are of help because they promote the flow of body fluids and loosen up stagnant material, thereby helping to carry off some of the toxic substances that have accumulated in the joint tissues. To obtain maximum benefits however, they must be carefully applied in accordance with the need of the individual case.

A Doctor's Drugless Remedy. Much trouble in arthritis centers in the lower back, in the lumbar region or in the sacroiliac joints. The solution to this trouble is in releasing the accumulated toxic irritants, in restoring free mobility and in strengthening the muscles that keep these joints in proper position. Skilfully applied manipulative techniques do much to loosen up the rigid and spastic joints of the back and help to strengthen and rebuild them.

However, since visiting a doctor's office is sometimes difficult or impractical, the exercises that I am presenting in this chapter, done carefully in one's own home, provide to a great degree the benefits that can be obtained from some of these treatments.

Physical Exercises Only One of Many Tools. Physical exercises and the various manipulative techniques that I am mentioning are of tremendous help in arthritis, but keep remembering that they represent merely one of the many tools that have to be employed if this painful affliction is to be overcome.

To really get well, you must in addition to the exercises, follow the overall health-building program that I describe in these pages. A carefully planned diet, an abundance of rest and sleep, the comfortable hot epsom salt baths, emotional control and peace of mind are essential parts of this overall health-building program and must be followed by the arthritis sufferer if he is to get well.

Patience Is Required. I keep emphasizing that we cannot wave a magic wand, and presto, the joint impairments or deformities disappear. The road to recovery is paved with patience and perseverance, and a well-planned regimen of natural care is essential if you are to succeed in getting well. The various exercises and manipulative techniques when correctly applied are of great help in arthritis, but never disregard the need of adopting a complete health-building program if you are to succeed in uprooting this difficult affliction. This program calls for drug elimination and adherence to a healthful living plan, plus all other drugless measures that provide relief of pain without any danger of complications or side effects.

Chapter Summary

1. Physical exercises and carefully applied manipulative techniques relieve congestion, promote drainage of toxic material and restore the flow of blood and the lymph fluids.
2. Exercise regularly to overcome aches and pains of arthritis-stiffened body parts.
3. Deep breathing exercises supply the body with oxygen and help cleanse out pocket sites of toxic waste accumulations.
4. "Loosening up" exercises are good for stiff limbs.
5. Physical exercises and the various manipulative techniques when carefully applied are of great help in arthritis, but always remember that they are merely part of a complete health-rebuilding program.

10

WHY ARTHRITIS
SUFFERERS REQUIRE MORE
SLEEP AND REST

Pains and stiffening of the joints put the arthritis sufferer's body under much internal tension. This tension drains vitality and aggravates the arthritis condition. Sleep and rest are essential if the circulatory system, the hormonal system, and the various vital organs of the body such as the heart, the lungs, the kidneys, and the liver, are to regain the necessary self-regenerative powers. While the arthritis sufferer needs to keep his body physically active to prevent the joints from becoming stiff and to overcome existing congestion, he must also be sure to obtain an abundance of sleep and rest to promote regeneration and rebuilding. Maintaining a balance between activities and rest is vital towards self-healing.

Rest Helps to Overcome Inflammation. An acutely inflamed joint must be favored. It needs rest, not forced activity. But the entire body, too, must be provided with sufficient rest and sleep so that it can recuperate and rebuild. A "localized rest" is provided when pressure and strain is kept off the inflamed joint or through the use of a temporary support, while an abundance of sleep and complete body rest helps to rebuild the health and strength of the whole body.

During rest and sleep, the body promotes its own drainage of congested fluids and helps to eliminate toxic waste products. This is especially the case when rest and sleep are part of an over-

all health-building program. When a joint is severely inflamed,
enforced exercises have to be suspended until the acute inflammation has either been overcome or is in the process of being broken
up. Let the flame "burn itself out" or "spend itself" by means of
rest, internal detoxification, and decongestion.

How to Provide "Rest" to an Inflamed Arthritic Joint. If your
knees, ankles or hips are acutely inflamed, see that these joints
get the rest they need by sparing them. Take your hot epsom salt
bath, and then apply a cold, moist compress over the inflamed
joint, but then remember the compress has to be well covered to
get warm. Or apply first a moist, hot compress and then follow
it with a moist, cold compress which is kept on until it gets really
warm, actually hot. Repeat this three times daily. Follow the previously outlined deep breathing exercises. You may exercise the
joints that are not acutely inflamed but be careful to avoid placing too much strain on the joints that are acutely inflamed.

The contrast temperature compresses help increase the flow of
blood and other body fluids to the inflamed joints and promote
drainage of congested material. This helps to reduce or overcome
swellings and congestion.

How Unnecessary Exertion May Increase Arthritis Distress

Enforced activity, pushing the joint to do more than it can
tolerate, often creates more inflammation. This should be kept
in mind when you suffer from any acute joint inflammation, and
it also holds true in an acute attack of sciatica. The sciatic nerve
is the largest nerve in the body and is composed of a multitude
of fibers which control the functions of the lower back and the
lower limbs, as well as some of the vital abdominal organs. An
acute sciatic attack may be brought on by inner emotional and
physical tensions, by internal toxemia, by disturbances in the
digestive or other internal organs, or by an arthritic condition
where deposits of calcium cause a distortion in the lower back
joints leading to pressure and inflammation of the sciatic nerve.

Our internal organs may be in poor health and yet we may not
be aware of it, since the nerves that control the functions of these
organs do not transmit the sensation of pain. The spinal nerves

that connect with these internal organs, however, often register the existing inner disturbances, and when these nerves become overtaxed or fail to receive the rest they need, it will often lead not only to an intensification of the arthritic pains, but intensify the existing internal disorders as well.

Rest Helps Detoxification. During the period of rest, the body's organs regain their strength and are enabled to carry out the various detoxifying processes that help to get the arthritis sufferer well. Rest helps to rebuild the functions of the colon, the kidneys, the liver, and the other organs of elimination and this helps to rid the body of accumulated toxic waste products.

Store Up Energy with Lots of Sleep. Even if you feel the need for 12, 14, or 16 hours sleep a day, don't fight it! You never sleep too much when your body needs rebuilding and strengthening. I don't want you to neglect your walks, your exercises, or the other care you need, but make sure to get all the sleep you can. As your body gets stronger your need for sleep will diminish and your exercises and other physical activities can then be increased.

Self-Help for Insomnia Problems. Many arthritis sufferers pay for their inside and outside tensions with sleeplessness. These tensions interfere with sound sleep. Insomnia can be overcome by adopting certain natural practices which induce a normal desire for sleep. Here are several measures that I have successfully employed to help arthritis sufferers overcome their insomnia and sleep more soundly:

1. Have your evening meal early, and keep it light. The all too common habit of working late, rushing home to a heavy meal, and then working all evening on some "homework," often leads to indigestion, tossing and turning, and frequent trips to the bathroom during the night. A light meal is easier for a tense stomach to digest. A glass of vegetable juice before bedtime will encourage relaxation and eventual sleep.

2. Always remember when sleeping and resting to choose the most comfortable position. Make sure your bed is comfortable and firm enough to encourage restful sleep. Avoid uncomfortable sleeping arrangements. To see whether your mattress is ample, measure yourself and then add 10 inches. The arthritis sufferer

needs a full-size mattress to allow for normal turning and comfortable arm and leg movements. For any man five-foot-ten or taller, this means at least an 80-inch mattress. Also, each sleeper in a bed needs at least 36 inches in the width of his bed for restful movement. If the arthritis sufferer does not have sufficient freedom of movement to alternately relax different sets of muscles, he awakens feeling cramped and tired.

3. Relax yourself in the evening. Don't overload your mind with thoughts about work. Keep away from arguments. Refuse to be drawn into any conflicts. Soft music, a pleasant book, simple meditation, will ease tensions.

4. Often, a walk will help relax that "tight" feeling. Walking of course, is a highly recommended exercise for arthritis sufferers. And while walking, do deep breathing! If the arthritis sufferer has a tendency to be lazy, having a dog would be of help. Everybody knows that a dog has to be taken out for a walk.

5. A soothing Sleep-Ease Tonic often helps to induce sleep. Here is a suggested tonic made of natural ingredients; it soothes the system while bathing the internal organs with a natural balm. Take carrots, celery, stringbeans, green peas, parsley, and any other green or root vegetable in season, add enough water to make a vegetable broth. Bring to a boil, then boil under a low flame until the vegetables are fully done. Take a cup of this beverage before retiring. Sip slowly; it is invigorating and relaxing.

6. The hot epsom salt baths taken before retiring often induce sleep in most cases of arthritis. Occasionally however, the hot epsom salt baths may be too stimulating and then this keeps the patient from falling asleep. When this is the case, my advice is that the bath be taken in the morning, but that immediately after the bath the patient return to bed for a period of rest and relaxation.

7. Cold feet interfere with sound sleep. Make sure that your feet are kept comfortably warm by using when necessary either a hot water bottle or a heating pad.

How to Make an All-Natural Hot Toddy Nightcap. Heat one glass of apple juice together with one tablespoon of lemon juice.

When the bubbles appear, remove from the flame, pour into a glass, then stir in a sprinkle of cinnamon for flavor. Stir vigorously and sip slowly. The minerals in the apple and lemon juice act as a soothing balm to the nerves and induce a natural sleep. The warmth helps ease tensions. This Hot Toddy Nightcap is All-Natural and most comforting.

Adopt The Sleep Habit. You can do this when you work at it consistently and it will make you tranquil and strong. Arrange to retire at a regular and decent hour. Learn to discard the problems of the day, and learn to dream or think pleasant and enjoyable thoughts. What a blessing if you can train yourself to float into pleasurable nothingness. It will induce relaxation and make you more contented and cheerful. It will help you digest your food, and will hasten recovery. Make the sleep habit a lifetime habit.

Sleep Is Nature's Tonic and Rebuilder. It strengthens your body, it gives you added vigor, and makes you get well much faster. Beware of sleeping pills. The sleep you get with them is *not real sleep.* To get well and strong we need *real sleep,* not sleep induced by drugs. We want real sleep, *not* false sleep; false sleep induced by sleeping pills provides only false hope and ruins our health only more.

Relaxed Life Speeds Arthritis Help. Haste wastes energy. To rebuild health, the arthritis sufferer must slow down, since speed interferes with recovery. To check haste, eat slowly, talk slowly, walk slowly, and even think slowly. Thinking slowly does not lessen your ability to think clearly; it actually makes you more alert. By thinking more slowly we check the crowding of thought upon thought and thus we are able to see everything in its proper perspective—and it also speeds up healing and repair!

Retire at Regular Hours. Establish a regular retiring schedule. Late TV and radio programs and exciting activities should be shunned. Late parties and activities that keep the mind and emotions overstimulated and overactive into the wee hours of the night should be eliminated.

When you feel sleepy, surrender to the Sandman. Your body is telling you that you need rest and sleep. Pay attention to it and be rewarded with more rapid healing of your arthritic condition.

How to Strike a Balance Between Rest and Sleep. The arthritic joint must not be abused or overworked. It should be kept active whenever possible, but without overstrain. To rest the tired or ailing joint, keep it free from physical strain. To sleep, the entire body should be fully relaxed for the night. You should also, whenever possible, take "rest breaks" during the day. A quick nap or just a little rest period by lying down in between tasks, can do wonders for you.

Self-Rehabilitation Program for Arthritis Sufferers. Complete inactivity forced upon arthritis sufferers can often lead to increased symptoms. Increased joint deformity, muscle atrophy, and general debility are often the outcome of enforced and prolonged rest when not needed. Many immovable arthritics show a variation of residual scars, badly deformed hands, an ankylosed hip or knee, a stiff back or general muscular atrophy.

Enforced inactivity often leads to a loss of calcium and phosphorus. That is why self-rehabilitation can be speeded up by alternating the position from supine to prone and lying first on one side and then on the other side.

In many cases it is advisable not to use pillows for sleep or to use only a small pillow since pillows push the head too far forward and warp the normal cervical curve. This is a matter for individual discretion though, since the patient's comfort is paramount and individual adjustments must be made.

Increased movement is possible with a walker, walking with a cane, stair climbing, bicycle riding. Often, occupational therapy is helpful. Exercises should be adopted to the need and the ability of the individual case. But never force, and never overdo.

Whenever possible, sleeping on the right side or on the abdomen is recommended. A position that many of my patients have found most comfortable and that I consider most beneficial when it can be adopted without strain, is lying on the right side with the right shoulder and arm backward so that the body's position is oblique or at a 45° angle. The body resting partly on the right side and partly on the abdomen, offers freedom from tension and induces an easy and restful sleep. Of course, this position is possible only where joint involvements allow it.

The Sleep-Inducing Plan That Helps My Patients Go to Bed Refreshed and Arise Refreshed

Make sure that your stomach is not overloaded. Do relaxing deep-breathing exercises. Take your hot epsom salt bath before retiring. Find your most comfortable position. Keep your feet warm. Be well covered; be careful not to use too heavy or too little covering.

In Some Cases Complete Bed Rest Is a Must! That is, until the agonizing pains and the severely acute inflammation has subsided or is less severe. This need is often essential in severe attacks of acute sciatica, in severe sacroiliac joint inflammation, in acute disc problems, or in other severely acute forms of arthritis attacks where the pains are excruciating and crippling.

How to Differentiate between Need for Rest and Need for Activity

Acutely inflamed or injured joints need rest. This gives them a chance to knit and heal. But it is also essential that the stagnant fluids be kept moving so that the congested and toxic material be carried off. That is why we have to plan a compromise program, a way of care that accomplishes both. When the joint is acutely inflamed and in agonizing pain, it needs rest, not motion. This is why we sometimes have to insist on complete bed rest, or in the case of a local joint problem, limited use of the affected joint.

At this moment, I am thinking of the time when I was called to see Lottie R. Lottie was an old friend of mine and while in New York she kept in close touch with me. But then she moved away and for years I didn't hear from her.

One morning, I received a call from her. She was very sick and needed help desperately. What happened? Awakening one morning, she found herself practically "paralyzed" from excruciating pains in her back which traveled down into her legs. The pains in her back and in her legs were so intense that any effort to move only brought on more agonizing pains. The pains were so agonizing that all she could do was scream. A neighbor hearing her screams broke into a window and came in to see what she could do to help. She then telephoned to Lottie's husband who had left earlier for work. She also called a doctor.

Arriving that evening in the city where she lived I found that Lottie was suffering from a very acute sacroiliac condition with a severe involvement of the sciatic nerve.

Just touching her lower back or the slightest movement was enough to make her scream from pain. It took her husband, her daughter and myself some time before we could get her into a hot epsom salt bath which gave her some soothing relief.

It was obvious that Mrs. R. needed complete bed rest. She couldn't have gotten out of bed if she had wanted to, and she was not the kind of person that ordinarily could be kept down.

She was kept in bed for several weeks. But she also had to get all other care that would help break up the existing inflammation and promote the drainage of the stagnant congested fluids that brought about her collapse. I first put her on a grapefruit juice diet. She stayed on this diet for three weeks. All she had was grapefruit about every two hours or whenever she desired it.

She also needed some exercises. But she couldn't move. So I got her started having her wiggle her toes several times a day, as well as doing some deep breathing exercises. Her husband was also instructed to turn her gently from side to side because lying in one position or on one side often leads to more stagnation and sometimes to pneumonia.

When the pains lessened, I had her start with the feet exercises, getting her to move her feet up and down, and then moving the ankles inward an outward.

She still was unable to get out of bed. The inflammation was still acute and had not yet cleared up sufficiently to make getting out of bed possible.

Later as the pains continued to diminish she was able to start with the leg raising exercises, raising first one leg three times, then the other leg three times, then both legs together three times.

Ultimately she was able to get out of bed, and in time was able to resume her normal activities. I wish to stress at this point that in these cases the patient must be especially careful not to start walking too soon, since pains can easily be reawakened.

This happened about 25 years ago. While visiting Miami recently I met Lottie again. She is now 75 years old, a vital, vibrant woman, belying her age in every way. At this time she was getting ready for an extensive trip abroad, and during all the years since that attack, never had a recurrence of any pain. The reason for it is obvious. Lottie adheres to this healthy way of living, and never deviates from it. She eats the best of natural foods, takes her daily walks, and exercises regularly. She knows there is no substitute for a clean, healthful way of living.

Immobilization of Acutely Inflamed Joint Sometimes Essential

In local acute joint swellings, rest to the acutely inflamed joint may be essential at times. Where this is the case, an ace bandage can be of great help. While the ace bandage is worn, the care that promotes detoxification and that rebuilds the general health of the body must be followed.

I have had many patients under my care who suffered from acute rheumatic swellings and stiffnesss in the knee, but who could not stay away from their daily work. They simply had to continue earning a living. How did I help them? I advised them to temporarily keep the acutely painful knee partially immobilized by using an ace bandage. This provided the needed relief from pain. Then by adhering to a complete health-rebuilding program, including those exercises that could be done, the acute rheumatic swellings were gradually overcome. This is the way acute pains are often made to subside, and the patient returns to better health. For further discussion of how to use the ace bandage, turn to Chapter 11.

Lila B.'s Fight against Sleep and Rest. In a previous chapter I describe the case of Lila B. who regained her health after suffering for years from arthritis and a number of other highly debilitating ills. Lila originally came to see me after having suffered for

years from severe low back pains as well as pains and aches in
other parts of her body. Recurrent gallbladder attacks and various
other digestive upsets were some of her other health problems.
She also suffered from migraine headaches and often complained
of a variety of nervous reactions. She was extremely debilitated
and greatly overweight.

I had no difficulty at first in getting Lila to rest. As a matter of
fact, a great deal of sleep and rest, a good diet, the hot epsom
salt baths, and a well-regulated program of exercises helped to
overcome practically all her physical ailments, and to a considerable degree helped her to develop an entirely new outlook on
life. Within about six months Lila was practically all better.

But after getting better, while still adhering closely to her diet
and all other health-maintaining instructions, the idea of continuing to get enough rest seemed to her a "waste of time." Lila had
a responsible position in a commercial educational enterprise,
had a home and two children to take care of, was interested in
her garden and insisted on working in it. She also took long walks
every day, attended various exercise classes, and often kept busy
into the wee hours of the night. Now, I have no objection to walking and exercising; as a matter of fact, I encourage it, but not at
the expense of rest and sleep. And so, while, because of her diet
and other good care, her physical disorders did not show any signs
of recurring, some of her nervous symptoms began popping up
all over again.

I insisted on the need for more rest, but Lila would not listen.
But there came a time when Lila could no longer continue, and
she was forced to do what I told her. And you should hear the
praises that she now sings—to rest and sleep; and see how happy
she is to be alive again!

Co-Relate Physical Activities with Rest and Sleep

In the preceding chapter I discussed the benefits that the arthritis sufferer can derive from physical exercises and various types
of manipulative treatments and gentle deep body massage. In this
chapter I stress the need for an abundance of rest and sleep.

All of these measures are of great help in arthritis. Active physical exercises and the various manipulative techniques benefit the arthritis sufferer because they improve the circulation of the blood and other body fluids, promote the drainage of congested and stagnant matter, loosen up stiffened and rigid joints, and restore greater flexibility and freedom of motion. But to overcome the arthritis condition, an abundance of sleep and rest is equally essential. This strengthens the body and helps to replenish the used-up reserves. To strengthen the body, to normalize its functions, and to aid it in its effort to restore itself to real health, an abundance of rest and sleep in addition to all other required care is a *must*!

Rest to the Internal Organs Helpful. I pointed out on previous occasions that periods of limited food intake or complete fasts are of great help in arthritis. They help because they promote the elimination of toxins and provide a great deal of rest to the internal organs and tissues of the body. Added to this however, the need for physical activities, as well as sufficient rest and sleep, must never be overlooked. Both physical activities and exercises as well as sleep and rest—physiological rest as well as physical rest—must be part of an overall health-rebuilding program if the arthritis sufferer is to get well.

Sleep Tips to Relieve Arthritic Distress

1. Sufficient rest and sleep are essential if body tension is to be overcome and pain is to be relieved.
2. For localized relief of an acutely inflamed joint, partial immobilization of the joint is often necessary.
3. To create a favorable atmosphere for sleep-inducement, follow the steps outlined in this chapter.
4. A Natural Hot Toddy is excellent for inducing sound sleep.
5. Note the special sleep-inducing plan that has helped many of my patients.
6. When complete bed rest to arthritic joints is a must, find out how you must proceed to control and overcome stagnation.

11

HINTS ON HELPFUL
MECHANICAL AIDS FOR
ARTHRITIS RELIEF

In my treatment of arthritis, the use of mechanical aids is sometimes unavoidable, and occasionally actually helpful. But when one of these aids is suggested to you, make sure that you really need it, and then use it only as long as it is actually necessary and no longer. Don't let it become a "habit," since this can only prolong the disease and at times even add to the disability.

THE COLLAR AROUND THE NECK

You undoubtedly have noticed the iron or plastic collars that some people wear around the neck. This device is often put on to relieve severe arthritis pains in the neck. It provides relief of pain because it keeps the neck warm and keeps it in one position; in other words immobilizes it. However, while providing relief of pain, this device, if worn too long, can give rise to a variety of problems. It often encourages the deposit of more calcium in the arthritic joints of the neck and in some cases may even lead to permanent rigidity and stiffening.

Rest and Warmth Helpful. It is true that warmth and immobilization of acutely inflamed joints often provide great relief of pain. However, since the device mentioned above often gives rise to unpredictable difficulties, I prefer that those who suffer

143

from acute arthritis pains in the neck obtain the help they need in other and safer ways.

A More Recent Innovation. One of the more recent devices used for patients suffering from severe arthritis in the neck is a cervical collar made out of foam rubber. This collar, while providing warmth to the neck and limiting its movement, does not completely immobilize it. Whenever warmth and a certain amount of rest to the neck is indicated, this type of collar could be used as a temporary expedient. This collar can be taken off or put on whenever desired. It can be used as a temporary measure when needed, but at no time should it be worn constantly or over an extended period of time.

Get Rid of Arthritis Pains While Getting Rid of Your Disease

Do everything possible to obtain relief of pain. But also do everything that is necessary to control or overcome your arthritis condition. This means not only resorting to aids that provide warmth and rest to the inflamed and acutely painful neck joints, but also adopting a program of care that detoxifies the body, carries off stagnant and congested material, and brings about the needed repair and healing. A flannel bandage snugly wrapped around the neck will often provide support and warmth to the painful neck joints, and is often a more desirable aid as a means of obtaining the needed relief from pain. Use it when necessary, but at the same time adhere to the program of care that eliminates the causes of the disease and uproots the affliction as far as possible.

Bed Rest and Soothing Warmth Sometimes Necessary

Where the pains in the neck are excruciating, putting the patient to bed for two or three days and applying a bag or a sock filled with heated salt or sand, often provides great help. This provides an even, soothing warmth, counteracts spasms, relieves contractions, and brings about the needed relief of pain. This is a much safer way of obtaining relief than through drugs and usually more beneficial, especially when it is used in combination with all the other care needed to counteract the disease and re-build the health of the patient.

After the acute pains in the neck have been sufficiently relieved, mild exercises are advised while the entire health-building pro-gram is continued. I have no objection to the metal or plastic device mentioned above when used in fractures since in these cases the broken parts have to be kept in place so that they can grow together. In arthritis, however, our aim should be to clear up the inflammation as rapidly as possible and then rebuild flexi-bility and freedom of motion. Using a device such as the iron or plastic collar for weeks and sometimes even months often leads to the deposit of more calcium in the joints, encourages more stiffening, and our aim to regain flexibility and freedom of motion is often defeated. While warmth and rest or partial immobilization may at times he necessary, this should be attained by either a warm bandage or complete bed rest and the applica-tion of heat as described above, and as soon as possible, gentle, mild exercises should be encouraged.

Benefits of an Elastic Bandage. In severe arthritis of the knee or ankle, an elastic bandage such as an ace bandage wrapped around the joint often provides great relief of pain. The elastic bandage rests the joint, keeps it warm, and helps relieve con-gestion. It should be put on cross-wise; it should be wound around the joint snugly and firmly to provide adequate support, but it should not be put on too tightly since we must be careful not to interfere with the circulation. A padding of cotton wadding placed underneath the bandage provides added warmth to the joint and is often of additional help.

Use with Caution. A bandage of this kind applied to the knee or ankle is often helpful in providing relief of pain, but make sure to remove it as soon as the acute pains have subsided. Gentle exer-cises and use of the joint should then be encouraged. Don't let the bandage become a permanent "crutch." The joint should be re-turned to free use as soon as possible to promote circulation and restore freedom of movement. And bear in mind that an elastic bandage worn temporarily to partially immobilize an inflamed and painful joint is infinitely more advisable than the use of a cast or a brace. While providing rest and warmth to the painful and inflamed joint, an elastic bandage carefully put on does not completely arrest the joint's movements and therefore does not encourage the development of rigidity and stiffness in the joint.

Support Sometimes Needed in Acute Pains of Upper Back. In arthritis of the upper part of the back, acute pains sometimes radiate into the rib cage and chest. In these cases, an elastic bandage wrapped around the upper part of the back and chest can be of great help since it limits the movements of the painful part and provides the needed rest and warmth. Here too, however, it should be used only as a temporary expedient and should be removed as soon as the pains have been relieved and the support is no longer necessary. Deep breathing and other gentle exercises are then started. These exercises should gradually be increased, but again remember the need for caution. At the slightest feeling of discomfort, discontinue the exercises and permit the painful part to rest.

Temporary Use of Belts for Lower Back Pains. I also do not obejct to the use of a temporary support for an acutely painful back. The severely irritated and inflamed joints in the back may cause increasing pain upon movement, and a belt may provide much needed relief. However, this too must not be relied upon as a permanent "crutch" since this in time could weaken the back even further. The reason for wearing a support is to protect the joint against excessive strain and friction and to give the body a chance to overcome the inflammation. As soon as the pains lessen, its use should be discontinued. Our goal is to rebuild the health of the back rather than make the wearing of a belt a permanent habit.

Overall Improvement of Health Necessary. Overweight, ptosis, (protruding large abdomen), and prolapsed organs also place a great strain on the back muscles and its joints, and cause severe back pains. The conditions that cause the added strain to the back must be corrected and the general health of the body must be rebuilt if this painful affliction is to be overcome.

Use of Joint Should Be Encouraged. In discussing bursitis I pointed out that those who suffer from an acute attack of bursitis in the shoulder should keep the arm of the painful shoulder in a sling, but that as soon as the acute pains have subsided the "climb the wall" exercises should be started. This restores movement in the joint, promotes better circulation, and prevents the joint from becoming stiff and rigid. In bursitis, this prevents the development of a "frozen shoulder." While an elastic bandage or some similar support may be necessary or even advisable to provide rest and warmth to a badly inflamed arthritis joint, it should be removed as soon as the acute inflammation is brought under control and the pains are relieved. The joints should then be used with gentle care, and exercises should gradually be introduced to strengthen and rebuild them.

TRACTION—ITS BENEFITS AND LIMITATIONS

Traction is often considered beneficial in certain forms of arthritis such as a disc problem or in any other form of degenerative joint disease, especially of the lower back, but how traction is applied often determines whether real benefits are obtained, or whether it creates only more damage. Traction when used correctly can help to loosen up stiffened and spastic joints, but when used the wrong way, it could actually lead to a more serious condition.

Mechanical Traction Often Increases Pain. Dorothy M. suffered from a severe degenerative joint disease in the lower part of her back. It all began from a severe injury to her spine some years back. The pains in the lower part of her back were agonizing. The only time she obtained relief from these pains was when she was lying on a hard floor! She also developed sciatica in the left leg with excruciating pains radiating into different parts of the leg. She became so disabled that she was taken to a hospital where she received the routine care applied in these cases. She was also kept in traction for two weeks "which was very painful." After the traction, Dorothy was worse than before.

Then she was brought to my office twice-a-week for treatments. The back seat of the car in which she was brought had to be fixed up like a bed to enable her to lie down and rest while traveling to and from my office. She was so badly crippled and so full of pains that when she first came to see me she was barely able to walk, shuffling her feet step by step, each step full of agony. It took six months of regular care before her severe back pains had completely cleared up. On the seventh month, she attended a family gathering and was able to dance like any normal person. Following her recovery, she was able to get back to her regular activities as well as helping her husband in his business, and since then has been more active than ever before without any recurrence of her pains.

How Dorothy Recovered. Where traction and pain-relieving drugs proved futile, a change to natural care not only corrected the damage in her back but also rebuilt the health of her whole body. This again is the secret that helps to get these patients well. Dorothy was given proper bed rest, comfortably hot baths, contrasting moist, hot and cold compresses, supervised exercises, plus the various manipulative treatments that improved the circulation to the damaged joints of the back. It promoted the elimination of stagnant material, and started her on the road to recovery.

Her diet consisted of raw fruits and raw vegetables with a minimum of cooked foods. No one single measure when used by itself is enough to do a complete job. However, when a complete program of care is adopted, and when it is consistently followed, success in the great majority of cases is inevitable.

Manual Traction Best

In telling of Dorothy's experience I do not wish to imply that traction is harmful. Traction has proven of great help in arthritis but generally the manual type of traction is best since in this type of traction the pull that is exerted can easily be controlled. Many of the exercises that are described in the chapter on exercises, as well as carefully applied manual manipulative treatments administered by a skilled osteopath, chiropractor or naturopathic physician, provide the type of manual traction which is of great help in painful arthritis of the back. These treatments as well as the exercises that I am presenting in this book, when carefully administered, help to loosen up tightened and spastic muscles, increase flexibility and motion, and bring about great relief of pain. On the other hand, the force employed with the conventional type of traction often causes only more damage to the diseased and crippled joints, and this often leads to more suffering and pain.

A Case of Damaged Hip Sockets

Sixty-eight-year-old Augusta W. has been a victim of arthritis for a great many years; the damage in her hip joints had already reached a point where the sockets of both hips, the hollow spaces in the hip bones to which the heads of the long bones of the thighs are attached, showed a tremendous amount of destruction. In fact the socket of the left hip had already become so badly eroded that the head of the long bone actually penetrated into the pelvis.

She found her way to our plan of total care, and X rays taken only five weeks later showed that within this relatively short period of time the badly eroded hip joints were beginning to fill in with new calcium, and that this provided a greater degree of stability and balance in her walking.

To the average layman, these early X-ray disclosures may not have been too significant, but if you give it some thought you soon begin to sense the miraculous power of nature, the power within our body which with the slightest encouragement starts healing and rebuilding. Before, the destruction in her hip sockets and in the other joints kept proceeding unmercifully, but providing the body with the right kind of help even for this short space of time proved sufficient to halt further destruction. What was even more significant, however, was that healthy calcium began to settle in the eaten away parts of the bones, and this proved how rapidly healing and repair can start when the body is provided with the right kind of care.

The Type of Mechanical Traction That Proved Helpful

Because of the deep damage in Augusta's hip joints we felt that some kind of mechanical traction could be of added help. But how were we to get the mechanical type of traction that would be safe? After careful deliberation we developed a device that can easily be put together in any home. We took a pair of shoes, and to each shoe attached a clamp. Then to each clamp we attached a fine, flexible wire. Metal cans, each of which was to hold about one or one-and-a-half pounds of sand or salt were then appended to the other ends of the wires. (These cans were to be filled with salt or sand or any other substances to the weight of one or one-and-a-half pounds). Then pulleys were attached to the foot of the bed over which the wires were to glide.

Augusta was put to bed, the shoes were put on her feet and while the wires with the filled cans were rolling over the pulleys, they exerted a mild pull or traction. She received this treatment twice daily, 30 to 45 minutes at a time, and the gentle pull of the weights exerted just enough traction to loosen up the spasms and the rigidity without causing any damage.

A Safe Homemade Traction Device

The reason this homemade traction device is superior to the conventionally used type of traction is because of the light weights. In the conventional type of traction, weights up to seven pounds or more are usually attached, and in some cases the amount of traction is actually intensified even more when straps are attached under the patient's arms or on the neck to augment the pull.

This simple home traction device can easily be put together. It can be put together in the average home, but it should be used only under careful supervision and only when actually needed. Where the foot of the bed is too low or does not lend itself to the attachment of pulleys, a rod run across the foot of the bed at a suitable height can easily serve the purpose.

Careful Traction, the Right Kind of Food, and Healthful Living Helped

When Mrs. W. arrived at our Spa, she used a walker. Each step was torture. But then only after about one week or two, she was able to discontinue the use of the walker and change over to the use of two canes. Later she managed to get around with only one cane. She began to take longer steps. Before leaving the Spa, although her short stay could hardly be considered as more than a bare beginning, she was already a much happier and more hopeful person. She dreaded the idea of ultimately landing in a wheelchair and of having to live out the rest of her years in it, and she was determined to continue with this type of care at home. It finally dawned on her that only by adhering consistently to this care will she succeed in restoring her health sufficiently to enable her to return to a more active and useful life.

A Manual Traction Technique

With the patient lying on the back on a couch or bed with firm support (as when a board is placed under the mattress), with the legs fully extended, the leg that is to be stretched is placed on the operator's shoulder and then slowly lifted as high as the patient's condition permits. Additional pressure applied on the patient's foot while holding the leg in this upright position provides additional traction. The pressure on the foot is then released and the leg gradually lowered. This form of traction repeated three or four times at a session helps to stretch the leg, releases spasms in the leg and in the lower part of the back, brings about greater flexibility and freedom of motion and provides significant relief of pain. It is usually a good policy to apply this type of traction first to one leg and then to the other. The results in most cases are most gratifying.

Why Braces and Casts or Splinting Should Be Avoided

Braces and casts are helpful in fractures where broken bones have to be properly aligned and given a chance to grow together and heal. But in arthritis it is best that they be avoided. When these devices are worn over an extended period of time, they often encourage the joints to grow together and permanent ankylosis will often set in. To get the arthritis patient well, our aim should be to overcome the acute inflammation of the joints and to promote as far as possible total repair and rehabilitation, not stiffening or immobility.

MRS. R.'s "PAIN-FREE ARTHRITIS" LED TO CRIPPLING AND LOSS OF POWER

Many cases of arthritis are pain-free and these cases are often of an insidious nature, since the disease keeps on progressing with little or no knowledge on the patient's part. Claire R., in her 40's, suffered from severe stiffness of her right leg with gradual loss of mobility. She suffered virtually none of the usual arthritis pains. At the time she came to my office for care, she had already been wearing a brace on the right foot for almost three years. She had no pain, but the ability to use the right leg had gradually but perceptibly been diminishing. It was like a creeping paralysis with progressive loss of power. A doctor told her that she would have to wear a brace for the rest of her life, and warned her that serious consequences would follow if she tried to get around without it.

When I saw Mrs. R., I felt confident that much could be done for her, and the X rays that she brought along only confirmed it. They disclosed the presence of extensive osteoarthritic changes in the joints of the spine, as well as a certain amount of osteoporosis, a demineralization of the bones which often shows up in cases of arthritis.

The Program That Helped Mrs. R. My first step in Mrs. R.'s case was to discard the use of the brace. To regain a certain amount of use of the right leg, the brace that prevented mobility had to be removed. I insisted that she try walking without the brace a little at a time, cautiously at first so as not to put too much strain on the greatly weakened and wasted leg. I also outlined a series of simple leg exercises to rebuild the wasted muscles and to strengthen them. Among the first exercises that I outlined for her were the simple leg exercises described in a previous chapter. She was to raise each leg slowly three times, and then both legs three times. I also suggested deep breathing exercises to promote more thorough oxygenation of the blood and tissues. Later we proceeded with feet, ankle and toe exercises. Because of the existing paralysis in the right leg, she could not at first do many of these exercises with the right leg. However, as her general health improved, she gradually regained a certain amount of use of the paralyzed leg and was able to use it in many ways impossible before.

Uric Acid Crystals Flushed Out. Since the accumulation of toxic wastes and uric acid crystals continues to worsen these cases, a detoxification program is essential. Mrs. R. was placed on a complete detoxifying program. For the first few days she abstained from all food, taking nothing but fresh water whenever she desired it. Then for two full days she was kept on a grapefruit juice diet. In those two days she drank freely of freshly pressed grapefruit juice whenever she felt hungry, but did not touch any other food. Then she followed with a diet composed of essential life and health-giving foods, the foods that I have enumerated in some of the previous chapters. A one-day complete fast or grapefruit juice diet was repeated weekly. She took hot epsom salt baths daily, and I insisted that she obtain much rest during the day and get a full night's sleep. All these changes helped to rebuild the overall health of her body, and in time restored a great deal of strength to her wasted and paralyzed muscles, and this ultimately brought back considerable use of the right leg.

Henry's Arthritis Made Him a Cripple. Henry M., unlike Mrs. R., did not wear a brace on his leg. But in all other respects, his case was very much similar. When coming to see me, he was hardly able to walk. He dragged one of his legs, walked with great difficulty, and felt greatly depressed, actually despondent. He had always been an active person and succeeded in building up a highly successful enterprise, and now that he was becoming constantly more crippled and losing the power to walk, he felt as if all life was coming to an end.

The paralysis in his case, too, was caused by softened and weakened bones (osteoporosis) in the spine shifting their position and leading to compression of certain nerves, thus bringing on a certain amount of paralysis in the leg. Tranquilizers, belladona, barbiturates and other drugs were prescribed for him for many years, but the more he continued with his drug taking, the greater became his crippling.

The Program That Helped Rebuild His Strength. In Henry M.'s case, too, I insisted that he discontinue all drugs. After keeping him for two days on a grapefruit diet to start the elimination of toxic wastes, I then followed up with a natural health-building food regimen. I insisted that he eliminate coffee, give up his before-dinner cocktail, that he avoid all seasoned foods, and that large raw vegetable salads, ample fresh fruits, moderate amounts of steamed vegetables and small amounts of easily digestible protein make up the bulk of his diet. One day a week he was to eat nothing but fresh fruit, and at least one or two other days a week he was to eat only fresh fruits all day until the evening, and then in the evening he was to have a large raw vegetable salad, a small amount of lean fish or chicken or any other easily digestible protein foods, and one or two steamed vegetables. He was also to adhere to a regular program of deep breathing and leg exercises, and to make sure to get enough sleep and rest.

Mr. M. has now been following this program for about five or six years and, while the paralysis in the affected leg has not been completely overcome, he has regained a considerable amount of strength and power in it. You don't see him dragging or shuffling his feet any more, and altogether he is a new, dynamic, vital person. He is continuing to follow this new way of living; in fact, by now he has adopted it as his permanent way of life. After regaining his strength, he threw himself into his business with renewed enthusiasm, and he often has remarked that he is able to do so much more than he did in the past because this care has made him so much stronger and healthier.

Osteoporosis Creeps Up Slowly and Insidiously. Osteoporosis, as I have explained before, is the opposite of thickening and hardening of the bones. In osteoporosis, the bones become porous and fragile and as a result can easily bend or fracture. In arthritis there is a derangement of calcium metabolism. In some cases an excess of calcium accumulates in the joints and they become thickened and stiffened, while in others the bones lose their calcium and other essential minerals and this makes them soft and fragile. When the bones lose essential minerals they can easily bend and often even fracture. In shifting their position, they often cause pressure on nerves and this leads to a certain amount of numbness, impairment of function, and sometimes even to a certain amount of paralysis.

Osteoporosis Sometimes Leads to Hip Fractures. When osteoporosis of the hip bones proceeds unchecked, it often leads to hip fractures. The typical hip fracture that occurs in old people is often due not to a fall, but rather to weakened and decalcified bone splintering and breaking and causing a fall. Neglected arthritis, where osteoporosis is present, can lead to such unexpected complications and this again should serve as a warning that the sooner proper care is provided in this bone- and joint-damaging disease, the better. And let us not delude ourselves by thinking that care is not necessary simply because there is no pain. Osteoporosis does not always give advance warning of its existence, and meanwhile bony destruction continues, causing more weakness and greater damage.

Home Remedies for Arthritic Relief

A Board Placed Under the Mattress Provides Firm Support. To provide firm support to your back place a board under the mattress. When resting or sleeping, lie flat on your back or find the most comfortable position. Provide your painful joints with enough support to make them comfortable but if at all possible, avoid using supports that arrest movement completely.

Use a Chair with a Firm Back and Firm Seat. Your hips and shoulders should be flat against the back of your chair. Do **not** sit in soft, overstuffed chairs or low chairs, which are bad for the arthritis sufferer's sitting posture.

When traveling in a car, use a back support to protect yourself against sloping. Firm back support will often make your trip in a car a pleasure instead of an ordeal.

Posture Pointers. Keep good posture whether in bed, sitting, standing, or walking. Stand tall. Keep your head up, chin in, shoulders relaxed. Knees and hips should be kept *comfortably* straight. Your weight should be kept evenly distributed on both feet. When walking, swing your arms easily at your sides. To step off or "push off," use the ball of your foot. Do *not* walk in a manner to suggest flat-footedness, shuffling, stiff-leggedness, or with your hips and knees bent.

Be Gentle with Yourself. Whether exercising or following any sport or physical undertaking, be gentle to your limbs. **Never** use force to straighten out a bent knee or any twisted and stiffened joint. **Never** try to force a spastic or thickened joint to a point where it causes severe pain. You will be able to move your joints much more freely and easily after you have loosened the attendant physical derangements that brought on the spasm or that caused the distortion. Be gentle. Avoid prolonged bending, avoid heavy lifting, avoid standing in one position or in one place for any prolonged period of time.

Review of Chapter Highlights

1. Mechanical aids should not serve as a "crutch" to replace use of a limb; rather, they should rest the affected joint and enable it to recover so that it can be returned to normal use.
2. An elastic bandage will help in many situations.
3. How to employ traction and manual manipulation safely and how to safely apply stretchings to loosen up stiff and spastic joints are fully described through actual case histories.
4. Follow suggestions for mechanical home traction where needed for painless relief.
5. Fasting, home traction, and manual manipulations are beneficial. They release acid crystals and toxic wastes, they help to restore better body functioning, and help rebuild the overall health of the arthritis sufferer.

12

A SEVEN-DAY PROGRAM TO
PROMOTE EFFECTIVE RESISTANCE TO
ARTHRITIC DETERIORATION

Before you commence with this program, keep this one point in mind: *You Must Not Expect the Impossible.* Just because you have decided to adopt a plan that has helped many thousands of arthritis sufferers and that if followed consistently and faithfully can help you, too, you must not assume that results can be attained quickly and effortlessly. It is not like waving a magic wand and presto—your health is back to normal as if no damage ever existed.

It is true that many patients obtain considerable improvement almost from the very beginning and that a great many regain their health within a relatively short period of time—four months, six months, or even a year.

Extensive Damage Requires More Time. On the other hand, where the disease has already progressed to the point where extensive damage has set in, much more time may be required before results are attained. It is also well to bear in mind that in some cases the damage may already have reached a point where complete restoration is no longer attainable. However, even in these cases the patient need not despair since intensive and persistent care in accordance with the principles outlined in this book most often provides significant and gratifying results. While the damage may have already reached a point where complete or total correction is no longer possible, persistent and thorough care can bring about sufficient improvement to help restore the patient to a useful and pain-free life.

Make Use of Your Potential Inner Healing Power. If you really wish to get well, remember that patience, perseverance, and close adherence to the plan I am outlining in this book will ultimately pay off. Whether your body can recover quickly or requires a great deal of time, the miraculous power of healing within your body, if provided with the needed help, will ultimately bring about a restoration of your health.

HIGHLIGHTS OF A SEVEN-DAY "START OFF" DIET

Each Case Is Different. Before going into a discussion of a Seven-Day "Start Off" program, let us bear in mind that no two cases are alike. People differ and the degree of damage in each case may also require certain individual adaptations. The Seven-Day "Start Off" Program that I here outline should therefore be regarded merely as an example of how you should go about getting started. The program that I am presenting in these pages and that I have used with phenomenal success in many thousands of cases shows you the path that you have to follow if you are to really get well.

How to Get Started

Whenever possible, the arthritis sufferer starts by taking just pure, clean water or freshly squeezed fruit juice for one to three days. Avoid fluoridated water. You can flavor the water with lemon juice and take a sip whenever hungry or thirsty, or take 8 ounces of your favorite fruit juice, such as apple juice, pineapple juice or any other favorite fruit juice, about every two to three hours or whenever hungry. Sip it slowly or take it with a spoon or through a straw or glass tube. Where this start seems too strenuous or difficult, I advise at first a diet of fresh fruit in season. Any one of the fresh fruits in season should be eaten whenever hungry, or about every two to three hours for about two to three days, and this is then followed with a diet of fresh fruit whenever hungry or about every two to three hours until evening, and a meal of raw vegetable salad, baked potatoes or a small portion of any lean fish, lean chicken or lean meat, and one steamed vegetable in the evening. When eating fruit, choose only fruits in season and eat only one kind of fruit at a time.

An Integrated Seven-Day "Start Off" Diet

Following this, you can adopt any of the diets outlined in the preceding chapters, or plan a diet that conforms to the following Seven-Day "Start Off" Diet Outline:

MONDAY:

Breakfast: Raw apple, very ripe banana and cup of alfalfa, camomile or any other bland herb tea, gently sweetened with honey. If hungry between meals, raw fresh fruit, fruit juice, herb tea, or vegetable broth is usually permitted.

Lunch: Raw vegetable salad of lettuce, cucumber, grated carrots and celery, other raw vegetables available in season, baked or boiled-in-jacket potatoes, and steamed stringbeans. Then stewed or soaked prunes for dessert. Never add sugar or sweetening to fruit.

Dinner: Raw vegetable salad of romaine lettuce, grated raw beets, grated parsnips, green or sweet red peppers, or other desirable raw vegetables available. Then natural brown rice, steamed sprouts, baked or raw sweet apple for dessert. (I repeat, never add sugar or sweetening to fruit).

TUESDAY:

Breakfast: Bunch of grapes, small portion of cheese such as cottage cheese, pot cheese, farmer cheese or the Italian cheese, ricotta, alfalfa or any other favorite herb tea, mildly sweetened with honey.

Lunch: Raw vegetable salad of chickory, escarole, grated carrots and radishes, or other available vegetables. Baked potatoes or baked yams or corn on the cob, ripe pear or blueberries or any stewed fruit for dessert. (No added sweetening).

Dinner: Raw vegetable salad of grated raw carrots, raw grated beets, cucumber, celery, other seasonal raw vegetables, natural brown rice, steamed or boiled artichokes, apple sauce made of sweet apples only. (No added sweetening).

WEDNESDAY:

Breakfast: Large portion of melon in season, ripe baked banana, glass of raw skimmed milk or any favorite herb tea slightly sweetened with honey.

Lunch: Raw vegetable salad of chickory, celery, watercress, and grated carrots, or other raw vegetables in season. Steamed young beans and broccoli, shredded raw sweet apple.

Dinner: Raw vegetable salad of grated cabbage, sweet peppers, celery, cucumber, or other raw vegetables desired. Then baked or boiled-in-jacket potatoes, and steamed eggplant, also baked or raw sweet apple or pear, if desired.

THURSDAY:

Breakfast: Grated and slightly heated raw apple, unprocessed brown rice, favorite herb tea sparingly sweetened with honey.

Lunch: Large fruit salad (any fresh fruits available in season) 4 to 5 ounces of any of the soft, bland cheeses, fresh fruit or any herb tea desired, sparingly honey-sweetened.

Dinner: Raw vegetable salad of diced celery, grated carrots, diced apple and raisins, corn on the cob, steamed onions and celery stewed or soaked prunes.

FRIDAY:

Breakfast: Stewed pears, 1 or 2 slices of whole wheat or whole rye toast or 3 to 4 Swedish rye or whole wheat wafers, a glass of skimmed raw milk or the honey-sweetened herb tea.

Lunch: Raw vegetable salad of cut-up spinach leaves, celery, raw grated beets, grated kohlrabi, or other available raw vegetables. Then vegetable stew of young peas, celery and carrots; sweet raw or baked apple or peaches.

Dinner: Raw vegetable salad of lettuce, green peppers, grated cabbage, grated carrots, or other available vegetables with small portion of lean fish or chicken or any other easily digestible protein food. Young tender stringbeans, fresh fruit compote (no sweetening).

SATURDAY:

Breakfast: Grated, raw sweet apple; slightly heated, natural brown rice, the honey-sweetened herb tea.

Lunch: Salad of diced celery, diced apples and pears, grapes, a few seedless raisins served on a bed of lettuce, soft cheese such as cottage cheese, pot cheese, farmer cheese or the Italian cheese, ricotta, melon in season.

Dinner: Raw vegetable salad of escarole, cucumber, radishes, and grated turnips, other raw vegetables available, with baked or boiled jacket potatoes, young green sweet peas, baked eggplant, shredded raw apple.

SUNDAY:

Breakfast: Bunch of grapes, very ripe banana, glass of raw skimmed milk or the honey-sweetened herb tea.

Lunch: Raw vegetable salad of grated carrots, shredded cabbage, diced celery, grated parsnips, watercress, other available vegetables, freshly prepared vegetable soup, slice of whole wheat toast or Swedish rye wafers. Baked apple or any stewed fruit (unsweetened).

Dinner: Raw vegetable salad of green lettuce, spinach leaves, grated turnips, grated beets, with baked potato, steamed kale or other steamed greens, apple sauce prepared from sweet apples (no additional sweetening).

The above diet is often most suitable for a start. It is not too rigid and gives the person who is not accustomed to dieting a chance to realize that although it is essential that the conventional unhealthy foods be given up, the diet outlined still provides ample nourishment and the meals are pleasurably satisfying. Coffee, tea, sugar, white bread and other white flour and white sugar products, the refined and processed cereals, cakes, pastries, cookies, ice cream, chocolate, spicy foods and foods that are rich in hard, hydrogenated fats such as margarine, butter, cream, fat meats, and the high-content fatty cheeses, should be entirely eliminated.

Points to Remember as Part of Your Overall Diet Plan

Whenever possible select organically grown fresh fruits and vegetables. These foods, obtainable in many health food stores, are best because they are unadulterated and have not been tampered with by present-day artificial food manufacturing practices. Organically grown fresh fruits and vegetables whenever available plus unfermented, unsweetened fruit and vegetable juices, fine aromatic herb teas, the finely tasting vegetable broth powders, the varied whole grain products, organically grown brown rice, and unprocessed and unpreserved packaged dry fruits provide valuable nutrients to the sufferer from arthritis and should be used as part of an overall healthful dietary program. Remember your dietary program calls for natural, unadulterated, wholesome foods, and where organically grown foods are available, they should be preferred.

Develop Corrective Eating Habits. *Do Not Overeat.* Food excess creates toxins and an overburdened digestion. Eat slowly. Eating too fast often leads to overeating. Chew your food thoroughly. Bolting down food without proper chewing will interfere with the digestion and cause excessive fermentation. *Eat Only When Hungry!* Do **not** eat when emotionally upset or disturbed; if you do, the food turns to poison and impairs your health.

Total Fast Days Helpful. Devote one or two days each week to total fasting or a raw fruit juice diet. Those who suffer from a difficult digestive porblem or a badly debilitated nervous system will do best to omit the use of the citrus fruit juices such as orange juice or grapefruit juice. They may at first have to rely on soft, bland nonfibrous foods, and when adopting a fruit juice diet, apple juice is usually best. And never take the juices chilled. A more liberal diet including raw fruits and raw vegetables is gradually introduced after the associated digestive problems have been overcome or brought under control.

An Alfalfa Seed Beverage Highly Recommended. A beverage that is most enjoyable and a great help in arthritis is the alfalfa seed broth. Add six teaspoonfuls of alfalfa seeds to one quart of water, let it stand over night. Then bring it to a boil. Let it boil for ten minutes; then continue to slow boil for another 15 minutes. Strain, cool, and gently sweeten with honey. Make sure that you use organically grown alfalfa seeds, seeds that have not been chemically treated. These seeds are available in all health food stores. Take this beverage three or more times a day.

Another Most Helpful Alfalfa Seed Beverage for Arthritis Sufferers. Take one pint of unpasteurized and unsterilized apple cider vinegar. Add enough unpasteurized and unsterilized honey to make a thick syrup. Pour the thick syrup into a bottle, and keep it under refrigeration. Before using, *always shake well.* Then take one tablespoon of this mixture in a glass of pure water—no fluoridated water, no chlorinated water, no distilled water, just good clean spring water. City dwellers can buy bottled spring water in drug stores or have it delivered to their homes by companies that specialize in supplying this kind of water. Add to it one heaping teaspoonful of *unheated* and *untreated* alfalfa powder (the whole alfalfa plant ground up); make sure that it is unheated and untreated. Stir vigorously and drink it. Take twice daily.

Note: Natural vinegar usually gets darker with age, but this should not worry you. If a sediment settles on the bottom of the container, do not discard it. Shake the bottle well to mix it. The sediment is the "mother" of vinegar, and is valuable. When the bottle is empty, make up the next batch in the same bottle without rinsing it.

Corrective Physical Exercises Part of the Integrated Health Plan. Corrective Physical Exercises Should Be Performed Daily: Read all the instructions in the preceding chapters that deal with the benefits corrective physical exercises provide in specific arthritis problems and apply them to your own individual needs. Remember to exercise slowly and rhythmically, and to rest after your exercises.

Above All, Develop Self-Understanding. Think what would happen if a train dispatcher would keep on transmitting in rapid succession contradictory orders over the wires. Confusion? Actually much worse: possibly total breakdown!

This is exactly what happens when your brain keeps transmitting conflicting messages to your digestive system or some of the other organs of your body. All the organs of the body are guided in their functions by the brain which transmits its messages by way of the nerves to each part of the body. When adverse influences cause upsets to the nervous system or bring on emotional upheavals, the various organs of the body pay for it in a number of ways. When this happens to the stomach, instead of eliminating the unholy or unwholesome influences that brought about a disruption in functioning, most people swallow a dose of some stomach-alkalizing remedy and think that they have helped themselves. The result is actually only more internal havoc and more intensive disease.

Most Bodily Functions Are Carried on by the Subconscious. This area of the brain usually works calmly and methodically, but when it becomes upset by any of the influences that impair the functions of the nervous system, discord begins to set in. Trembling of the body, nervous indigestion, irregular heart action, and a variety of other disturbances begin to show up. It also manifests itself in more severe arthritis symptoms. Always remember emotions and arthritis often go together. And this also holds true about inner tensions.

Destructive Emotions Upset Digestion and Foment Arthritis

Peace of mind is vital. Nervous tension impairs digestion, and improperly assimilated food leads to nutritional deficiencies. This can aggravate arthritis and create only more suffering.

Nervous disorders are due to many factors. Fatigue, wear and tear, varied adverse influences such as drugs, chemicals, coffee, liquor and sweets, often disrupt nerve functioning and lead to emotional discord.

Never Permit Anger to Take Over. "Anger is the wind that blows out the light of reason." I do not recollect who said it, but it is well that we keep this point in mind when we feel like getting angry. Anger distorts vision, equilibrium and understanding. Whenever anger hits, remember composure, calmness and patience are your best medicine. Sometimes the fact that you can keep calm under stress may annoy those who try to use you as a sounding board, but don't let this upset you! Adhere to your determination to keep calm and serene, since this ultimately shows how foolish and destructive anger can be and how much better it is to keep calm and composed. Contemplation, reflection, plus a natural healthful way of living, pave the way for calmness, serenity, and a new and more composed life.

Sugars, ice cream, pies, pastries and cookies overstimulate the body and make one more irritable and excited. These so called foods, "empty foods" as they are often called, are not vital foods and make a person only more nervous and restless. They also rob the body of essential food elements and contribute to much disease and suffering.

To help conquer arthritis, the sufferer from this disease must avoid all destructive emotions and adopt an attitude towards the problems of life that is both constructive and protective.

Naps and Rest Periods Are Helpful. If you can take a daily nap or rest period at a convenient time of the day, you will do much to develop relaxation and this will be of great help in overcoming your arthritis condition. A businessman who cannot find the time to "let go" because he is too busy can still do much for himself by using this "Jiffy Relaxation" program.

Sit back in your chair. Close your eyes. Let go completely. Focus your mind on a clear, blue sky. Think of absolutely nothing except the clear blue sky. Let your body go limp, part by part. Let yourself go. . . .

This "Jiffy Relaxation" program takes just five minutes but if followed a few times a day, can produce most gratifying results. *Remember:* Close out all unpleasant or disturbing thoughts and replace them with thoughts of beauty, kindness, composure, patience, tolerance. Get yourself into a peaceful and relaxed frame of mind. Think of the happiness that you can create for yourself as well as bring to others. Think of a pleasant vacation or an enjoyable trip that you would like to take; shift your thoughts to something pleasant and constructive, and what a blessing it will be to you and to those around you.

How Nancy Created a New Life for Herself

As an example of what a healthier frame of mind can accomplish for you, let's take the case of Nancy M., age 56, suffering from severe arthritis pains. Her back, her hands, her knees, her neck, her shoulders were constantly full of pain. After becoming acquainted with Nancy's condition I soon realized that while her arthritis would be amenable to care, I would not succeed in getting her well unless I succeeded in getting her to gain control of her emotional instabilities and fears. Nancy, the wife of a minister, was engaged in many church activities and her relations with some of the members of the congregation contributed much to her state of unhappiness, her conflicts, and her feelings of insecurity. I made her realize that the grass is not always greener on the other side of the fence, that we all have our problems, and that, while living, problems will always be with us.

However, the great majority of problems that arise in our day-to-day living are not life-threatening, and can easily be handled when we develop a calm and more serene outlook on life and restore ourselves to a state of physical and emotional well-being.

Nancy Was Considerably Overweight. At the start I made sure that Nancy realized the importance of adopting a well-planned dietary program. I placed her at first on an exclusive fresh fruit diet. She was to eat only one kind of fruit whenever hungry or about every two to three hours until evening. For the evening meal she was permitted a large raw vegetable salad, baked potatoes one day or a small portion of lean fish or chicken on alternate days, and one or two steamed vegetables. Baked apple or any stewed fruit was optional, if still hungry. She was to use no butter, salt, or any of the sharp irritating spices, and add no sugar to her fruit. Later other foods were permitted, but essentially she was kept on a wholesome, healthful diet conforming to the ideas that I am describing in this book.

Then I Insisted on Ample Sleep and Rest. She was instructed to take a nap or a rest period every afternoon and to learn how to let go, how to relax. Deep breathing exercises and the knowledge that at last she was on the road to better health helped to accomplish much of this.

I also encouraged her to adopt a program of regular body-building exercises. For her back and abdominal muscles she was instructed to do her leg raising exercises, and for the severe pains in her neck she was to rotate her neck and bend it from side to side every morning and night. All these exercises are fully described in the chapter on exercises.

I also instructed her to take her comfortably hot bath every night before retiring, and then to retire immediately.

Looking over the notes that I made when she first came to see me, I find that aside from suffering from arthritis all over her body and being extremely nervous and distraught, she also had difficulty in digesting her food, suffered from cystitis (a very annoying bladder disorder) and severe headaches. Now her arthritis pains are practically all gone, she has no difficulty in digesting her food, her bladder condition and her headaches have long cleared up; and nothing could now drag her back to her previous unhealthy habits of living.

Marital Problems Increase Arthritic Attack. There are situations in which family hostility and destructive emotions such as anger, jealousy, hate and envy cause psychosomatic upsets and increase arthritic symptoms. Many patients I have treated proved that emotional explosions or frustrations in the home often cause an intensification of arthritis symptoms. Often these frustrations are actually only a matter of our own outlook on life, of our inability to cope with the problems that face us, which we then take out on ourselves and others. Don't block your road to recovery by failing to make the needed emotional adjustments. It is interesting to note that men who suffer from arthritis are not as emotion-prone as women, although men are not exempt.

How to Obtain Release from Nagging Problems That Undermine Normal Body Functioning

There have been many times when nervous or hysterical patients would call me in the middle of the night and hysterically complain about feeling chilly and stiff all over, and this often happens with patients who suffer from only a minimal amount of arthritis. What do I usually tell these patients? "Get into a comfortably hot bath for a few minutes, use a hot water bottle to your feet to make sure that your feet are kept warm, do some deep breathing exercises, and go back to sleep." And as an after-thought I sometimes tell these patients, "Learn to relax, keep warm, and be at ease, for tomorrow is a new day, a better day, a more beautiful day."

Most often these patients would call me the next day to tell me that they had followed my advice, that after doing what I suggested to them, they fell into a sound sleep and awakened the next morning much refreshed and relieved. They considered it all so marvelous although what I had told them to do was surprisingly simple.

Program to Cope with Psychosomatic-Induced Arthritis

1. *Train Yourself to Be Relaxed and to See Many Sides of Life.*

2. *Learn to Dwell on the Sunnier Side of Life.*

3. *Slow Down and Learn to Be at Ease.*

4. *Follow the Good Way of Living: Discard ALL That Is Harmful and Destructive to Your Health.*

Establish Your Own Creed of Life. A set of rules that one of my patients adopted as a guide to a good way of living is worth emulating. These are the rules that she lived by:

1. *Keep Healthy the Natural Way.* Why the natural way? Because this is the only way of getting well and keeping well. Good food, fresh air, sunshine, physical exercises, an abundance of rest and sleep, creative work, and a calm and serene outlook on life are the foundation stones upon which good health is always built.

2. *Be Constructive and Positive in Action and Thought.* We either tear down or build up; she preferred to build up.

3. *Be Ever Ready to Learn.* None of us possesses all the wisdom, all the knowledge; the more we are willing to learn, the more we gain in stature and strength.

4. *Add to Growth and Development.* Unfoldment, growth, ideas and thoughts help to enrich our life and make us more creative human beings.

A Thumbnail Program for Growth and Development

1. Adopt a more positive outlook on life.

2. Rebuild your capacity for seeing good and discarding evil. We create much of our inner toxins and our deep sufferings by the way we think and the way we feel. We have the capacity to alter our attitude towards people and towards life, and by making a real effort to uncover the good qualities in other people we create for ourselves a richer and more contented life.

3. Become an open channel for the inflow and outflow of love, kindness and compassion. Let these feelings radiate to others, and you will soon find that a great many of your nervous troubles will fade away. As you rid yourself of destructive emotions, so do you also rid yourself of acid wastes and many pains and aches. You ease psychosomatic tensions and help restore normal body balance.

In telling you how to go about adjusting your way of thinking, I don't mean to imply that by doing this all your problems will automatically disappear. Life always presents us with a variety of problems, but when we follow a program of living that keeps us in a healthy condition, we gain the strength and maturity that enable us to face these problems and cope with them.

Mrs. S., one of my most recent patients, is a case in point. Mrs. S. placed herself under my care suffering severely from arthritis pains all over her back. Since we are the product of many influences, I don't as a rule stress only one phase of my plan but insist that a fully integrated program of care be adopted. But in Mrs. S.'s case, her emotional problems were so overwhelming that in addition to stressing the need for adopting a good nutritional program and a healthy way of living, I also placed special emphasis on the need for developing a more serene and constructive outlook on life. I was fortunate in being able to get her to work with me, and as a result a most miraculous change has taken place in her body within this short time. Her arthritis pains have almost completely cleared up. When she started treatment, the skin on one part of her back was as hard and tough as leather and her muscles were stiff and brittle, but you should see how soft and pliable both her skin and muscles have become. Her joints are much more flexible and free, she is able to get a good night's sleep without resorting to sleeping pills, and she has become a completely transformed person.

Do Not Expect Miracles Overnight

In this chapter I have given you an outline of how you should go about starting your health-rebuilding program. Remember, this is but the beginning. Rebuilding the health of the arthritis sufferer often requires a great deal of time and patience, and the length of time that it takes to get well depends on a variety of factors. The degree of damage, the recuperative powers of the individual, and the persistence with which the program is followed, all have a bearing. Adopt this program, follow it consistently, give yourself the time it requires, whether it be a few weeks, a few months, a year or two years or even longer if necessary, since this is the only way you can succeed in uprooting your arthritis problem. Remember, you are the *master;* and if you adopt this plan and adhere to it faithfully and loyally, you will never regret it. It may take time, it may require patience, but the compensation that ultimately follows repays you for your efforts in an infinite number of ways. You are the only one that can determine whether you are to get well or continue to permit your arthritis to make deeper inroads into your body. And even where complete restoration is no longer possible, keep remembering that you are the one that can determine whether you rebuild your health to the maximum degree possible or whether the disease continues to make deeper inroads. So get on the bandwagon! Know what you are aiming for and keep at it.

Success Depends upon Faithfulness. Whether you follow this program under professional guidance or do it on your own, devotion to the plan is a **must.** Whenever possible obtain skilled professional help; this makes the task so much easier and you are much more certain of obtaining maximum benefits. However, where for one reason or another skilled professional help in natural healing is not within your reach, remember that *you* are still the **master,** and that after all is said and done *you still have to do the major part of the work* if you are to succeed in regaining your health.

A 79-Year-Old Socialite Gets Rid of Her Arthritis by Following This Program. Countless letters from arthritis sufferers from all walks of life have told of similar experiences. One of the letters that I found most fascinating was written by a 79-year-old socialite Mrs. H. H. W. After asking whether I was the doctor who recommended this natural health-building regimen for arthritis sufferers, she then continued: "Assuming that you are the same doctor, you may be interested to know that a year ago last July I was practically ossified after several years of arthritis, although I spent thousands of dollars on treatments by the most eminent doctors; but now after faithfully following the regime you laid down, my joints are again fine and I am almost entirely cured. I am really a living confirmation of your theory."

She then went on to say that her doctor in Washington approved of trying it "as he had done all that modern medical science knew about, without permanent relief."

She then concluded, "As I am nearly 79, I feel that my cure has been really phenomenal."

What About Smoking?

I haven't said anything in this book about the effect of smoking on arthritis. At this time there should be no need for me to point out how harmful smoking can be to our health. Its effect on the lungs has been amply publicized. Lung cancer and bronchial emphysema are increasing at an enormous rate in those who smoke, but its injurious effect does not limit itself merely to the lungs and the bronchial tubes.

Studies by the United States Public Health Service disclose that smoking increases the demand of the heart for oxygen while reducing the ability of the blood to supply it. Certain substances inhaled when smoking raise the level of fats in the blood, making it flow more sluggishly. Smoking also causes blood platelets to become "sticky" which increases the tendency towards clotting. Finally it raises the carbon monoxide in the blood, reducing the supply of oxygen to the heart, a condition that often leads to fatal heart attacks.

This highly placed government agency disclosed that a man between 25 to 35 who smokes two packs a day shortens his life-span by eight years, while one who smokes less than half a pack shortens his life by four years. I know that many people would rather shorten their life than give up smoking, but when you think of the agony and suffering of the diseases that are caused by smoking, then the picture is entirely different. It is not that you are merely shortening your life, but the years that you do live are filled with suffering and pain. Since one of the major factors in arthritis is an impaired circulation to the joints—a condition where the blood cannot carry enough oxygen to the joints and cannot carry off all its toxic waste products—it should be obvious that if the arthritis sufferer is to get well, giving up smoking is **essential.** Smoking impairs the metabolism of the body, distorts functioning, and if not given up, interferes with recovery.

Program Points of This Chapter

1. Set yourself a goal to follow: Proper diet, corrective exercises, sufficient rest, peace of mind and emotional control. A seven-day plan that can mean the start of a new life and renewed health.
2. Emotional control is often the key to solving the arthritis problem. How to adopt a more constructive attitude to rid yourself of destructive thoughts and the poisons they create is described in this chapter.
3. Benefits of relaxing to ease tensions are enumerated.
4. A program to cope with psychosomatic-induced arthritis is set forth.

13

THE ROLE OF VITAMINS
AND OTHER FOOD SUPPLEMENTS IN
FIGHTING ARTHRITIS

Have you ever wondered whether vitamins are food or medicine? If you obtain your vitamins from natural food sources, from the greens, from plant life, then it is a food. If you swallow vitamins that have been chemically produced, synthetic vitamins, then you are swallowing chemicals, drugs! Real vitamins are foods, while synthetic vitamins, chemically produced, are drugs.

Vitamins Merely One Part of the Whole Food Package

The discovery of vitamins contributed greatly to our knowledge of nutrition. This, however, must not overshadow the fact that vitamins are only one of many elements that our foods must provide if we are to be well nourished.

Vitamins Do Not Stand Alone. Vitamins are essential, but equally essential to good nutrition are minerals, enzymes, proteins, and a variety of other food elements, including elements that undoubtedly exist in food but have not as yet been isolated.

Take Foods Whole. If we are to benefit from vitamins we must get them in combination with all the other food elements as they exist in nature. Vitamins, minerals, enzymes, proteins, and other essential elements co-exist, and if we are to obtain real benefit from them, we must take them together—in one package!

This Means: No Isolated Vitamins. Remember, vitamins do not stand alone, they are part of the whole food package. To

supply what we need we have to take all that belongs in the package—not just vitamin A or B or C or K or P; and when we take
minerals, not just iron or calcium or potassium or any other
mineral separately; but all vitamins, all minerals, all enzymes,
and all other food elements as they come to us in food as it is
produced in Nature.

Deficiencies Exist. Of course, the sick and even many of those
who think they are well but actually are on the border line of
disease suffer from many deficiencies in vitamins, minerals, protein and other vital food elements. These deficiencies exist because
of our unnatural food habits and also because many of us have
undermined our ability to utilize the food we eat. Will we make
up for these deficiencies by taking one or even several of the many
food elements we need? Of course not! We must get all the vitamins, all the minerals, as well as all the other food elements we
need as part of the whole package of whole foods. We must
derive our vitamins, minerals, proteins, and all the other food
elements that we need for complete nutrition from natural food
sources.

This Means: No Single Element. To get well and then to make
sure that you keep well, you must get all your vitamins, all your
minerals, all your enzymes, all other essential food needs *together*
as they come to us in their natural form; better yet, as they are
derived from the greens and/or all-natural plant life.

This Also Means: No Synthetic Vitamins. Why no synthetic
vitamins? Because synthetic vitamins are not foods, but chemicals. They do not possess the spark of life and we are deluding
ourselves when we think that they can serve the same purpose
as the vitamins that we find in food as part of the whole package
of foods, the whole foods, the LIVE, VITAL foods!

All Food Substances Are Interdependent

When we speak of vitamins, remember that we speak of food,
not chemicals or drugs. People take vitamins because they think
that their food is lacking in certain basic food elements, and they
hope to obtain what the food fails to provide by taking specific

vitamins or supplements. All food elements, all the vitamins, minerals, enzymes, protein, and other essential food elements, are interdependent in their action.

In nature, food is balanced. It provides all the elements in varying degrees in balanced form. So when you feel that you are unable to obtain all the nutrients you need from the foods you eat, and you think you have to turn to certain supplements to make up for it, make sure that what you take is derived from natural food sources and provides all the elements as they are found in nature in their balanced and fully integrated form.

Get Acquainted with Your Health Food Store. The conscientious health food storekeeper and those who work in these stores can be of service to you in selecting healthful foods that provide whole, vital nourishment. Don't hesitate to discuss your needs with them.

Find an All-Natural Organic Food Supply Source. In this era, with an infinite number of life-endangering chemicals being used in agriculture and in food processing, you would do well to turn whenever possible to All-Natural organic foods. These foods unfortunately are not always available and not obtainable everywhere, but whenever you can obtain them, use them in preference to those that are grown the conventional way with artificial fertilizers and the use of chemical pesticides.

Chemistry has enriched man's life in an infinite number of ways and has made life more beautiful, but it has also given us many things that play havoc with our health or that delude us by making us believe that we get the real thing when in reality we get a mere second-grade product. See to it that you provide yourself with all the nutrients you need for healthful living and health rebuilding, and do not let yourself be fooled by imitations. Get all your vitamins, all your minerals, all your essential nutrients from natural food sources, not from the chemist's laboratory.

How Nutrients Repair Ravages of Arthritis. The nutrients needed to rebuild the health of the arthritis sufferer are available in abundance everywhere. They are in the greens, in the fresh fruits, in the luscious berries in season, in fact in all plant life. These foods, taken in their whole and natural form, provide the cells, the bones and the blood with all the body-building elements they need, and when our body suffers from certain basic deficiencies they help to supply our needs and get us well. Today, we know that all vitamins, minerals, amino acids, unsaturated fatty acids, enzymes, and other basic food elements work together to create internal healing and repair of arthritis-ravaged joints and systems. The aim of the arthritis sufferer therefore should be to obtain all these food elements in their most complete and *natural* form.

Deficiencies Have to Be Overcome for Recovery. Those who have made a close study of the subject know that arthritis sufferers are deficient in essential food elements. Vitamins A, the B-complex, C and D, are notably low in those who suffer from arthritis. Minerals, enzymes, amino acids, and other essential nutrient elements are also needed to rebuild and repair body tissues, body cells and bones, as well as the internal organs. All of these elements are often lacking in one way or another in the body of the arthritis victim. Like the weakened link in a chain, the absence or deficiency of one element leads to a weakness in the entire structure. The arthritis sufferer must make sure to use only those food substances that rebuild his digestion and that provide all the nutrients he needs.

Fresh Fruit and Vegetable Juices. One of the most valuable sources of vital nutrients is fresh fruit and vegetable juices. They supercharge the body with blood-building minerals, skin-building vitamins, digestion-improving enzymes, bone-nourishing protein, and are of inestimable value to arthritis sufferers. If possible, make your own juices at home. One of the best health investments is a fruit and vegetable juicer. These juicers are also obtainable in any health or specialty food store. Select ripe fresh fruits and vegetables. Favor those that are grown under ideal organic conditions, since they are most valuable from the standpoint of health and nutrition. Bottled juices may be used if freshly squeezed juices are unavailable.

Fresh Juices and Selected Natural All-Food Products Are Part of a Sound Health-Building Program

Juices and All-Natural health food products provide vital health-building elements but must not be regarded as possessing miraculous healing powers. Healing originates from within the arthritis sufferer's own body. Make sure that you provide your body with the raw materials it needs to enable it to bring about the necessary rebuilding and healing. Then see to it that you obtain all the other care such as the needed rest, the physical exercises, the special baths, and the specialized physical movements that will help loosen up spastic and rigid muscles and joints. And never forget what a sound mental attitude and proper emotional control can do for you. All this care plus good wholesome nutrition helps to put the arthritis sufferer on the road to recovery.

Live Foods Provide Healthful Living. The arthritis sufferer must live on LIVE, VITAL foods. The foods he eats must be vital, natural foods. Get the best foods available; these foods plus all other care outlined in these pages are your best medicine. If you are unsure what foods are best for you, don't hesitate to discuss your problem with a doctor or a practitioner who has made a thorough study of nutrition and who possesses a thorough knowledge of the principles of natural healing. Remember, no synthetic vitamins, no synthetic, processed or adulterated food products. They do not provide the nourishment you need and can actually interfere with your recovery.

Dr. Joseph Evers, a well-known German physician, made this point most explicit when in essence he stated: Take the most luxurious, the most festive meal, bury it in the soil, and what happens? It rots! On the other hand, take a single kernel of a grain and bury it in the soil and what happens? It multiplies 20 to 30 fold. Take a cooked or baked apple and bury it in the soil. Again it rots. But take a raw apple and bury it and you have an entirely different picture. It grows into a mighty tree that provides you with a constant supply of apples for years to come. This essentially makes the difference between LIVE, VITAL foods and foods in which the life principle has already been destroyed.

While vitamins, minerals, enzymes, protein and other essential food elements are needed, get them from Natural, LIVE, VITAL food sources, not in synthetic form.

Highlights of This Chapter

1. Nutrients help repair arthritic ravages by rebuilding bones, cells, tissues, glands and the bloodstream.
2. Obtain all your nutrients from natural food sources. Use the natural raw vegetable juices.
3. All synthetic or chemically produced vitamins and supplements should be rejected in favor of vitamins and other food elements obtained in their most complete form from natural food sources.

14

HOW TO HANDLE THE
INTERMEDIATE STAGES OF RECOVERY
FROM ARTHRITIS

Sufferers from arthritis seldom get well without going through a series of intermediate reactions because recovery is not in a "straight line." If you wish to know what really happens during these acute reactions, imagine yourself taking a trip on the high seas with high winds or with a storm tossing the boat up and down. The trip, even though the boat is traveling in the right direction, can nevertheless be most unpleasant. Restoring the body of the arthritis sufferer to renewed health is also not smooth sailing. The reactions that occur when changes are taking place and when toxins are being eliminated are often unpredictable and, just like the winds on the high seas, can be most disturbing unless we understand what is taking place and know what we have to do to ease the distress.

Reactions Are Beneficial. When handled correctly these reactions actually serve a beneficial purpose. They occur because the body is trying to uproot the disease and pave the way for recovery. They indicate that certain self-cleansing changes are taking place within the body, and while painful or disturbing when they occur, if cared for in the right way, they ultimately lead to renewed health.

Reactions a Sign of Toxic Drainage. In the handling of arthritis, one of your major steps is to promote the elimination of toxins within your body. The reactions that show up while the body gets

179

rid of toxins are symptomatic of this form of drainage. When toxins are being uprooted, they usually are not eliminated without some sort of visible signs or outward manifestations. These signs or symptoms are Nature's way of telling us that an upheaval is taking place in the system as a means of cleansing out toxic accumulations. If you understand what is going on at such times and give yourself the right kind of care, renewed health ultimately follows.

Typical Symptoms During Toxic Drainage

In many cases the pains from toxic drainage may become increasingly more acute, and often keep shifting from one joint to another. Occasionally the swelling in the joints increases, and fever either general or local, often accompanies these reactions. Various skin disorders such as boils, blemishes, eruptions and sores, and such other disorders as cramps, diarrhea, dizziness, headaches, nausea, extreme fatigue and restlessness, are some of the reactions that may show up as part of the curative process.

Expect Normal Crises. It is natural to become frightened when these unforeseen or unpredictable reactions occur, but when you know what they mean, you will not let them upset you. Get to realize that these reactions are to be expected, and when they occur know what you must do to overcome them in the quickest and most thorough way. The rest then follows, and before long you begin to note that you are really on the road to recovery.

Sudden Flare-Ups of Pain. During these acute curative stages, not only does more intensified pain show up in the joints that were painful before, but pains sometimes show up in joints that in the past have never been known to be painful. Arthritis is often present in joints even though they are free from pain. It exists in a dormant state, and while the body is uprooting its overall arthritis condition, a flare-up in these joints can sometimes be most surprising and even frightening. But once you understand what these flare-ups mean, you will put up with them, and before long you will be much the better for it.

Fever a Healthful Sign. Fever is one of the symptoms that often show up during an acute reaction, either generalized fever affecting the whole body or localized fever showing up in the affected joint or in some other part of the body. Most people fear fever. They think it a sign of ill health. Actually, fever is one of the body's defensive actions, and when it is taken care of in accordance with the program that I am outlining in this book, it only leads to better health. Fever develops when the body seeks to combat unhealthy or uncongenial influences. Normal body temperature is the temperature that the body maintains under normal condition. Increased temperature, as well as other abnormal symptoms, shows up when the body's healing powers are endeavoring to overcome an existing abnormal condition; in the process, these healing powers intensify certain bodily functions such as pain, pressure, inflammation, or bring about an increase in bodily temperature. The various symptoms that show up at such times such as fever, acute pains, redness and swelling, show that the body's healing forces are endeavoring to counteract an existing abnormal condition in an attempt to make the necessary adjustments and reestablish a better state of health.

Reactions May Be Brief or Prolonged. Arthritis recovery cannot be brought about overnight. There are no "instant" techniques. Some get well sooner, some may take a much longer period of time, and patience and perseverance are winning attributes. You are only short-changing yourself when you become impatient or lose courage when the going gets tough or more difficult. How often are reactions to be expected and how long will they last before final recovery sets in? That depends to a great degree upon the amount of damage and your body's own recuperative powers, as well as the complications that may have developed as a result of previous drug therapy. Fortunately, in most cases, the body's inner healing and recuperative powers can still be reawakened, and when properly directed, they ultimately lead to renewed health.

Recurrences Are to Be Expected. Reactions may recur at different intervals and often express themselves in different ways, not only in renewed joint pains but also in upheavals in other body organs. But no matter in what form they show up, whether in the form of joint pains, nausea, headaches, dizziness, digestive upsets, diarrhea, fever or outbreaks on the skin, remember this is merely Nature's way of telling you that the body is carrying out a new housecleaning job, clearing away the debris and preparing the body for ultimate recovery. Retained poisons or health-destructive elements have loosened up from their imprisoned confines and are being eliminated.

Why These Different Reactions? The poisons, the accumulated toxins, have to be eliminated, and when they start coming out, you can never tell where the effects may be felt. Then pain, swelling, tension, various symptoms of ill health, begin to show up or become intensified, and they continue until this phase of body "housecleaning" has been completed. This is then usually followed by a higher level of health.

Don't Get Frightened when Feeling Weak. Any of the disorders mentioned above and numerous others may show up as part of the body housecleaning process and should be recognized as serving a constructive purpose. In addition to the various disorders that show up during the curative phase, some who adopt our health plan may also feel extremely weakened and "depleted." When this happens some become greatly frightened because they think that this feeling of weakness is a sign that they are not getting the nourishment they need.

Actually this is not the case. The sense of weakness that shows up during the early stages of this care merely discloses how greatly depleted the body has become. Since our dietary program eliminates all overstimulating foods and beverages, the sufferer from arthritis suddenly finds out how weakened and depleted his body really is, and this only proves how essential it is to omit all body-depleting influences and adopt a plan of care that rebuilds the health and strength of the whole body.

Weight Loss Beneficial. This natural health-building plan inevitably causes a loss of weight. Those who are overweight are naturally happy about this loss. Those who are underweight on the other hand are often concerned. They do not realize that what is important is not how much they weigh but how healthy they are. During the process of detoxification, unhealthy tissues and toxic accumulations are being broken down and eliminated.

Swelling, thickenings, excessive deposits of calcium must be cleared away, and this usually leads to a loss of weight, whether overweight or underweight. The overweight usually lose a great deal of weight, but even those who are underweight will at first lose some weight. The body has to rid itself of undesirable and toxic substances, and this at first causes a loss of weight. Ultimately the overweight person attains normal weight, and the underweight one, even though losing weight at first, ultimately regains healthy and natural weight.

Drugs Defeat Our Purpose. Drugs that inhibit fever or suppress any of the other symptoms that show up during the curative reactions often only build other serious health problems. While suppressing the fever or any of the other symptoms, they often actually interfere with body elimination and ultimately only create a more severe arthritis problem. Our major aim at all times should be to rid the body of its unhealthy waste products, and when this is accomplished the acute disorders disappear of their own accord.

How to Make the Most of Fever. To *cooperate* with fever, start with complete bed rest. All solid foods should be stopped until the temperature returns to normal. When necessary, the warm cleansing enema should be used daily. Also make use of the comfortably hot epsom salt baths which should immediately be followed by a return to bed.

Obtain Experienced Help. Since cases differ, you should whenever possible obtain the help of a doctor or a practitioner who specializes in natural healing and who possesses the necessary skill and experience to guide you. In addition to such help—or in its absence—the arthritis sufferer must make sure that the plan of care outlined in this book is consistently and carefully followed.

How Mrs. I. "Cooperated" with Her Reactions. I am thinking of Olga E. I. whose case history I presented in a earlier chapter. While following her health program, Mrs. I.'s legs became flaming red, swollen and painful. The skin on both legs broke out in a deep red rash. This signified that "internal cleansing" was taking place. It showed that the body had succeeded in uprooting toxins that had to be eliminated and that, at that particular time, were being eliminated in a more intensive form through the skin of her legs. By placing her on a complete grapefruit juice diet for about a week or ten days and applying the rest of my detoxification program in a more intensified form, the swelling and the eruptions on the legs quickly cleared up, and following this she found that her arthritis condition had greatly improved and before very long had completely cleared up.

A Breast Lump Disappeared when Arthritis Was Cleared Up. When Katherine H. came to see me she complained of chest and back pains, and since she had a lump in one of her breasts she thought that her pains were caused by the lump in the breast. She gave a history of various allergies and was greatly frightened because she thought that the lump might be cancerous.

Upon examination I found that her pains were caused not by the lump in the breast but by arthritis. The lump in the breast was a condition that is found in many women when the glands in the breast become thickened and hardened. This condition is known as mastitis and is most often nonmalignant. By placing Katherine on a detoxifying program, by using the cleansing hot epsom salt baths, by keeping her on a healthful dietary program, and by getting her to adhere to her exercises regularly, I was able to help her in clearing up her arthritis entirely. The lump in her breast too began to shrink and in time disappeared, while her allergies have long since become a thing of the past. Yes, it took about a year or longer before Katherine H. recovered, and during this year she went through a series of reactions that ranged from painful rheumatic attacks to various respiratory reactions, but today she is completely freed from all these unhealthy conditions.

In her case, one of the most annoying reactions that showed up about eight months after she started with this care, was a skin eruption which appeared on different parts of her body. She was greatly disturbed. She thought that she had already become completely well and that this was an entirely new ailment. Actually, this was but a final "mopping up" of the toxic accumulations that the body still had to eliminate. Again she started on an intensified cleansing routine. Within about three or four weeks, her skin eruption had entirely cleared up and she was again her usual self, only healthier, more spry, more vital, freed not only from her arthritis but also from all the other disorders that plagued her in the past.

Reactions Must Be Met with Courage. When these reactions occur they must be met with courage and faith, they must be cared for in accordance with the principles outlined in this book. Avoid relapsing into former habits not conducive to good health; these only undo all the good you have done and bring about a return of many of your previous problems. These reactions are spontaneous responses on the part of the body's own healing powers in its endeavor to restore itself to health.

A PARTICULARLY DIFFICULT CASE HANDLED SUCCESSFULLY

Elizabeth C.'s was one of the most difficult cases that I have ever handled during my many years of practice. When she first started under my care about a year and a half ago, her legs, her hips, her shoulders, her wrists, her hands, as well as the lower and upper parts of her back, were badly crippled, enlarged and thickened. Each knee was heavily impacted with calcium and was almost three times its normal size. The right knee was barely movable, and when I tried to move it, it was excruciatingly painful, while the left knee, equally as painful and thickened, could not be moved at all. At the beginning I could not help wondering whether this knee had not already become completely ossified, in which case restoration of movements could no longer be expected. However, when some of the calcium began to dissolve and the knee began to return to its more normal size, it gradually started to loosen up and then slowly she was able to start moving it. By then I began to feel confident that with time the impacted calcium in the knee and in the other impacted joints would continue to loosen up further and that ultimately she would continue to regain more motion and with it a lessening of pain.

Her wrists, too, were swollen, locked and painful, but in time they too regained much of their flexibility and became almost entirely pain-free. Similar changes took place in her shoulders which were badly hunched over, locked in one position and extremely painful but now are freely movable and without any pain.

At first her pains were so intense that she could not find a position in which to rest. It took about three months before her restlessness and irritability began to diminish. By then, her appetite started to come back. She began to enjoy the food she was eating, and her sleep became sound and restful. With time the swelling and thickening of her joints kept on decreasing and with this her pains too began to lessen, although recurring healing reactions which appeared periodically brought acute pain.

Common Sense About Anemia. The presence of anemia in arthritis is proof that existing toxemia has impaired the blood-making functions of the body. A detoxification program, which is then followed by a diet of tissue- and blood-building raw, natural foods, usually overcomes the ordinary type of anemia within a short period of time. Ridding the body of its sediments and toxic wastes, then feeding it with LIVE, VITAL, easily digested foods, and providing it with the rest and care it needs restores the red and white blood cells to a healthy and vigorous state, which in time helps to overcome this disabling disease.

To help Mrs. C. whose case history I describe above overcome her anemia, I first made sure that she adopt a carefully regulated dietary program which included an abundance of raw vegetables and lots of greens. The green leafy vegetables grown under the rays of the sun and loaded with chlorophyl, give a healthful boost to the body. She was to take daily three to four cups of the alfalfa seed beverage that I described in another chapter of this book. I also advised her to buy a sturdy juicer, one that could extract the juices from the root vegetables as well as from the leafy vegetables, and take six to eight ounces of carrot, celery and parsley juice, or any other combination of raw vegetable juices two or three times a day between meals. As soon as the warm weather permitted, I urged her to expose her body to the healing and warming rays of the sun. She was to start first with ten minutes on each side, but then gradually increase her exposure until she was able to take one full hour at a time. She was instructed to take her sunbaths during the early morning hours or late afternoons when the sun was warm and comfortable but not too hot. She was warned to make sure not to overexpose herself to sunshine.

Because she was so badly crippled, Mrs. C. could not get into a bath tub and therefore had to take daily hot mustard foot baths, but later as her joints became more flexible and free she was able to get into a tub and then started to take her epsom salt baths. She also kept up with her daily exercises which were increased as her joints became more limber and pliable.

Mrs. C.'s Most Dramatic Reaction. However, before Mrs. C. reached this present state of improvement, her skin, too, like the skin of some other patients, broke out in a heavy rash. As if out of a clear sky, the skin on her entire back and chest, as well as other parts of her body, became extremely itchy, inflamed and covered with many eruptions. Ugly sores developed on her cheeks and face, and her lips became heavily covered with thick scabs. All this took several weeks to heal. But then miracle of miracles. As the skin condition cleared up, Mrs. C. became entirely free from pain. She was able to return to her work and now is an entirely new person.

This type of reaction often shows up when the body in its effort to rid itself of toxins uses the skin as its outlet. We can never predict how the body will rid itself of its toxins, but when during one of these reactions unexpected skin eruptions show up we must understand what it signifies and realize that it is but one of nature's ways of ridding the body of its toxins. At such time, all we need to do is but intensify the detoxification program by abstaining from food entirely or follow an exclusive juice or fruit diet for a few days and also follow through with all the other care that hastens the elimination of toxins through the other channels of elimination, and thus hasten recovery.

Let Reactions Run Their Course. Bear in mind what these reactions mean and make sure that you "cooperate" with Nature by letting them run their course, even though they are accompanied by pain or discomfort. Reactions should never be suppressed but helped along to their culmination through the use of the various health-restorative, pain-relieving, and comfort-providing measures outlined in this book. Let me repeat a sound warning: Do NOT try to suppress them since this only bottles up the disease and usually only creates a more serious arthritis condition. Drug taking lessens the body's ability to bring about the needed cleansing as well as the required repair and recuperation. Your aim is to clean out the disease-producing toxins and bring about a restoration of normal bodily functioning since this is essential if health is to be rebuilt. And when the body attempts to do a thorough housecleaning job, keep remembering that this is a beginning to ultimate recovery, and all you have to do to obtain the desired results is cooperate with it.

Main Points in Review

1. During recovery, healing crises are unavoidable. They are signs that the healing powers of the body are endeavoring to cast out toxic causes of the disease.
2. Recovery may be swift or more gradual depending upon the severity of the condition and the ability of the body to respond. Symptoms, too, may be mild or pronounced.
3. Weight loss is often a key to arthritis healing. Follow the plan outlined in this book and you will ultimately attain the weight that is normal for you.
4. Fever helps to cleanse your bloodstream and tissues.
5. Shun drugs since they bottle up the toxic body wastes and eventually lead to more suffering and greater arthritis damage.

15

HELPFUL HINTS
FOR HEALTHFUL EATING
AWAY FROM HOME

When away from home the arthritis sufferer must make sure to adhere as closely as possible to the same pattern of eating that he follows at home under his curative diet. The practices outlined in this book should be followed as closely as possible when eating in restaurants, at friends' homes, or under any other circumstances. A simple guide is to select foods in their most natural state and eat them in their most healthful form. Establish a healthful diet pattern, build it into your overall health restoration plan, and benefits will gradually begin to show up.

How to Meet the Food Problem when Away from Home. There may be times when you have to eat away from home. Be prepared and plan ahead. Use the same wisdom in selection as you would if you were in your own home. Even when you have to pass along a counter of foods that are yours for the taking, remember that *simplicity* and *natural* are your key guides. Since health-building foods are necessary for health rebuilding, you will more readily eradicate your arthritis by selecting healthful meals, whether at home or away.

How to Select Healthful Foods when Dining Out. When you choose a good restaurant, you should have no difficulty in ordering wholesome health-giving dishes. Pass up those sloppy, cooked-to-death abominations, and order what you know is best for you. You may want to be like your friends. That is, you may not wish to appear different. But who can object to your having a lettuce and tomato salad or a fresh fruit salad with some cottage cheese when lunching with a friend or business associate? A dish of seasonal berries or a fruit juice drink can round out the meal. This is sensible eating and should not raise eyebrows.

For dinner, a raw vegetable salad with a baked potato and a steamed vegetable, or a raw vegetable salad with some lean fish or chicken and some fruit for dessert certainly makes a nice, wholesome meal.

It is quite satisfying and just a good intelligent way of eating. As a dessert, any fresh fruit in season will do.

Alright to Order a Cocktail? When a friend or business associate orders a cocktail, so can you! Just order a glass of tomato juice, or your favorite fruit juice, or a mixed vegetable cocktail.

If the question should come up, just say, "Doctor's orders," and leave it at that. Or you may say that you just don't feel like a drink at this moment. This too works!

When invited to a friend's home for dinner, you need not make yourself conspicuous by any special diet. To begin with, you could have dinner at home and arrange to visit your friend after meal time. Or if this is not convenient, you can still use the same "Doctor's orders" explanation. In many instances, you will find your friend understanding and cooperative when you politely decline dishes that are not on your list and adhere only to the fresh fruits and vegetables and the lean meat, fish or poultry. Always eat moderately when eating away from home to be on the safe side.

How to Keep Healthy While on a Trip. When you travel, you can always select good food. It is possible to order fresh fruits and raw vegetables almost anywhere. This, plus a small portion of your favorite protein food as a main dish (meat, fish, poultry, cheese) prepared in a simple manner, or a baked potato or corn on the cob whenever available, makes a most desirable meal. When you follow this program, it is easy to keep healthy while on a trip.

Advance Planning Is Helpful. When having dinner alone or with friends in a restaurant, always choose an eating place that renders good service for you. Sometimes a little advance planning helps. You should get to know the restaurants that are cooperative in health diet matters. Or you may telephone ahead of time and arrange with the owner or maître d' for the special type of natural food you wish to be served. You can always arrange for a raw vegetable salad—with no dressing or a dressing that is good for you. If you desire, ask for sliced lemon to be served on the side. You can then squeeze the lemon juice yourself for a piquant flavoring on vegetables.

Select Plain Foods. To obtain maximum benefit from the food you eat, choose those foods that are as natural as possible, with a minimum of distortion. Prepared foods such as patties, soups, stews, certain mixed, chopped or diced salads (such as egg salad, fish salad, etc.) are disguised to create synthetic taste sensations. Select foods that are plain.

How to Eat When on a Long Airplane Trip. When we plan an airplane trip, I usually call the airline in advance and ask them to serve us fresh seasonal fruits—these could be grapes, apples, pears, peaches, and the like. I also request a ripe avocado or ripe bananas or some ricotta cheese, cottage cheese, or any of the other soft cheeses. This provides us with a most luscious and enjoyable meal, which is certainly much more gratifying and healthful than the conventional meals served on these trips.

Select Simplicity. The arthritis sufferer will rebuild and retain his precious health if simplicity in the choice of foods is his watchword. Food selection and combination should be simple! You would do well to have this in mind before you sit down at any restaurant table with a big appetite.

Keep Your Aim in Mind

Your major aim is to uproot your disease and rebuild your health. Any time you take liberties with your diet you only put another road block in your way. Nothing is worth the pain, the suffering and the crippling that bad living has created for you and that you will continue to create if you persist in eating food that is not suitable for you. Choose the best foods possible, plan a well integrated, healthful way of living, make use of the constructive health-restorative measures I am suggesting in this book, and you will be on the road to a newer and healthier life.

Summary

1. Food is the foundation for the restoration of health. Select natural, simple foods when eating at home or when away from home.
2. Plan ahead when dining out and arrange for natural foods to be served to you.
3. Keep healthy when on a trip by ordering natural foods.
4. Never apologize or be on the defensive. You have nothing to be apologetic about, you have learned what is best for you and you should be proud of it. If an explanation is ever necessary you can always say "Doctor's orders" or "I like it best this way."
5. Always remember your major aim is to regain your health and you only cheat yourself when you fail to do what is best for you.

16

RECIPES AND GUIDE TO
BEST MEALS AND BEVERAGES FOR
THE ARTHRITIS VICTIM

In planning your meals always remember that first and foremost come your *raw foods*. Raw fruits and raw vegetables are rich in vitamins, minerals and enzymes, as well as the essential trace elements needed for complete nutrition. Raw foods also provide protein in the finest and most natural form. A raw vegetable salad should be the major part of your meal at least once or even twice a day. Of course, those who for one reason or another cannot handle raw vegetables and fruits may at first have to adopt a soft bland diet, but they should at the same time resort to the type of care that will help them overcome the condition that is making the use of raw foods difficult or impossible.

Make Your Raw Vegetable Salad the Number One Dish. The primary dish should be a raw vegetable salad; add to it your favorite easily digestible carbohydrate or starch food or a small portion of one of the easily digestible protein foods. Among the best starch foods for the arthritis sufferer are potatoes baked or boiled in the jacket, yams, sweet potatoes, corn on the cob and natural brown rice.

Sweet Corn on the Cob Raw. Almost everybody loves sweet corn on the cob. When in season and when freshly picked, *raw, sweet corn on the cob* contains a wealth of precious nutrients and digestible starch in natural balance. Try eating it raw, and it will be a most enjoyable taste-treat.

Suggested Protein Foods. Among the wholesome protein foods are some of the soft bland cheeses, cottage cheese, pot cheese, farmer cheese, the Italian ricotta cheese and soybeans—also small portions of lean fish or lean chicken or any lean meat for those who feel the need for these foods. Nuts and seeds such as almonds, walnuts, sunflower seeds and pumpkin seeds, are excellent sources of protein but should be used sparingly since they are high in fat.

Non-Meat Program Most Healthful for the Arthritis Sufferer. From study and observation as well as from a lifetime of experience with patients and myself, I am convinced that for good health a well-regulated, well-planned non-meat regimen is vastly superior to one which includes the use of meat. A carefully regulated non-meat diet, followed consistently as part of a well-planned overall healthful way of living is the only sure way of building superior health, renewed youthfulness, and longevity.

Giving Up Meat Helpful but Not Essential. However, while giving up the use of meat can be of great help, this is not absolutely essential. When you include meat in your diet, make sure that you use an abundance of raw vegetables with it. My aim in this book is to explain how you can regain your health, and even if you cannot abstain from meat entirely, you need not feel that your case is hopeless provided you eat it in small amounts and in combination with a plentiful supply of raw vegetables and fresh fruits. In eating any food, remember that the less heat-processed the food (baked, boiled or broiled), the better.

How to Stay Young at 72, 82, 92, or Even 102. We have become so conditioned to anticipating old age with its debilities and crippling that we often regard them as inevitable. But this need not happen if you follow the program that I am presenting in this book and that has helped countless thousands of arthritis sufferers to renewed health and youthfulness. You are a child of Nature and if you work in harmony with Nature, renewed health can be yours.

Many people develop so-called "old-age" debilities at a relatively early age. Some who are only in the 40's or 50's or even younger are already old and decrepid looking, and this only because of their wrong-living habits which hasten decay, breakdown and premature aging. If you give yourself care in accordance with sound, healthful living principles, you will not only overcome your arthritis, but you will also rebuild the health of your entire body and gain renewed youthfulness, vigor, strength, endurance and an entirely new life.

YOUR RECIPES FOR HEALTH

Now that you have come to understand how essential good food and healthful living habits are for those who wish to eradicate their arthritis and gain renewed health and youthfulness, I shall present in the next several pages a number of healthful and enjoyable recipes that will prove how adequate and pleasing the meals can be that the arthritis sufferer is to eat to help him rebuild his health.

Vital Health-Building Raw Vegetable and Fruit Salads

SALAD SUPREME

3 carrots, medium size, 2 beets, medium size,
¼ head cabbage, medium size, ¼ lb. spinach,
1 large onion, 1 green pepper, 2 tomatoes,
6 radishes, 1 small avocado.

Dice onions in separate dish. Add soybean oil or any other vegetable oil. Cover dish tightly and let stand in refrigerator for one to two hours. Grate carrots, beets and cabbage; cut spinach fine and place each vegetable in separate mounds.
Add the diced onion to each vegetable mound. Cut green peppers into strips, slice tomatoes and use whole radishes for garnishing. Add slices of avocado. Use lemon juice or lemon juice and honey dressing if desired. Serves three.

RAW VEGETABLE SALAD
(A health stimulating meal)

3 leaves of Romaine Lettuce, cut up (diced), ½ finely grated small beet, 1 finely grated medium-sized carrot, ¼ finely grated cucumber, ½ cup finely grated red cabbage, 1 stalk celery, ¼

cut up onion, ½ avocado mashed in—Mix all ingredients together and serve with baked white potatoes, baked sweet potatoes, yams, corn on the cob, or your favorite protein. Optional, one steamed vegetable and baked apple, or any stewed raw fruit. Serves one.

A COLORFUL HEALTH SALAD

1 beet, ¼ lb. cabbage, ¼ avocado (in season)
or 2 tbs. cottage or pot cheese, 1 carrot,
1 stalk celery with tops, parsley (to flavor).

Mix finely grated beet, carrot and shredded cabbage. Add diced or cut up celery and parsley and serve with avocado (mashed) or cheese.

Serve with or without desired dressing. Serves one.

RELISH SALAD

2 cups finely chopped cabbage, 1 grated
onion, ½ cup chopped cooked beets, 1 cup
minced celery, 3 tbs. minced pimento, ½
minced green pepper.

Mix with tomato juice dressing or other favorite dressing. Serves two.

ROOT VEGETABLE SALAD

2 raw carrots, 2 raw beets, 2 raw parsnips,
¼ of a raw turnip, ¼ of a raw white potato,
1 baked sweet potato, ½ ripe avocado.

Formula—Grate the raw vegetables, mash the sweet potato in the raw vegetables. Use unsalted vegetable broth flavoring.

RAINBOW SALAD

3 carrots, 2 beets, 1 large yellow turnip
1 large or two small cucumbers, 1 bunch
red radishes, ½ cup fresh watercress or parsley.

Finely shred and mix carrots, beets and turnips. Place mixture on bed of watercress. Surround with sliced cucumber and red radishes. Season with lemon juice, oil and honey or other favorite dressing. Serves four.

MARINATED SALAD

1 small green cabbage (shredded), 2 cups shredded or grated carrots, 1 green pepper (diced), 1 cucumber (diced).

Prepare dressing: one cup equal portions of lemon juice, oil and honey, and pour over salad. Cover and place in refrigerator for one hour before serving. Serve on green lettuce leaves. Serves two or three.

GREEN SALAD

1 cup chopped dandelion leaves, 1 cup chopped chickory or Chinese cabbage, ½ head chopped green lettuce, ½ cup chopped spinach, ½ cup chopped watercress.

Mix all vegetables together and serve with lemon juice and honey or yogurt. Serves four.

EGGPLANT SALAD

1 good-sized eggplant, 2 stalks green celery, 2 large or 3 small green peppers, 2 medium onions.

Bake eggplant in skin. Peel and mash in wooden bowl with wooden spoon. Chop celery, peppers and onions, add to eggplant and mix thoroughly. Caution: Use wooden spoon to prevent eggplant from turning black. Serve on lettuce leaves. For dressing add lemon or lime juice. Serve with a baked potato. It makes a fine quick meal. Serves four.

GREEN PEA SALAD

1 cup fresh raw or steamed green peas, 2 stalks green celery, 1 heart of green celery, 1 medium or 2 small onions or some fresh scallions, 1 green pepper, 2 small ripe tomatoes.

Dice stalk and heart of celery, onions (or scallions), pepper and tomatoes. Mix together and add green peas. Serve on lettuce leaves. Your favorite nut butter dissolved with lemon juice makes a fine dressing. Serves two.

POTATO SALAD

2 lbs. boiled potatoes, 1 large green pepper,
3 stalks celery, ¾ cup finely cut parsley,
2 medium carrots, 1 large onion.

Peel potatoes and cut into cubes. Grate vegetables. Mix vegetables with potatoes. Make dressing of 2 tablespoons yogurt or soured milk, ½ ripe mashed avocado and juice of ½ lemon. Mix dressing thoroughly and pour over potato salad. Mix again and let stand in refrigerator for at least one hour before serving. Remove from refrigerator ½ hour before serving to remove the chill. Serves four.

FAVORITE SALAD

½ head fresh cabbage, 2 carrots, 1 green
pepper, 1 stalk celery, 1 onion.

Grate cabbage and carrots. Dice pepper, celery, onion and mix all vegetables together. May be served with lemon juice. Serves two.

CUT-UP SALAD

1 small head fresh green lettuce, 4 ripe
tomatoes, 1 green pepper, 1 large onion,
1 medium cucumber, 1 cup fresh crisp spinach,
a few sprigs of fresh watercress or parsley.

Cut lettuce into quarters. Cut up rest of ingredients and mix. Serve on beet leaves with sprig of watercress or parsley. Season with fresh lime or lemon juice or your favorite dressing. Serves four.

TASTY SALAD

1 cup shredded cabbage, 1 grated carrot,
6 green ripe olives (obtainable in health food stores),

1 clove of garlic, ½ cup diced green pepper,
½ cup diced celery.

Soak olives in plain water for ½ hour or longer to remove salt.
Rub a clove of garlic on salad bowl and toss in all the vegetables.
Cut in olives and mix well. Add your favorite dressing. Serves
two.

APPLE VEGETABLE SALAD

2 apples, 4 scallions, 2 stalks celery, 16 spinach
leaves.

Chop vegetables, shred apples and mix. Serve with eggless mayon-
naise or choose your favorite dressing. Serves two.

HOT WEATHER SALAD

1 cup dandelion leaves, 1 medium or 2 small
onions, 2 ripe tomatoes.

Chop together and serve on crisp green lettuce leaves. Add some
cottage cheese or avocado and your favorite dressing. Serves two.

REFRESHING SALAD

¼ medium head green crisp cabbage, 1 medium
or 2 small beets, 2 small carrots, 2 ripe
tomatoes, 1 medium cucumber or 2 small ones,
1 medium green pepper.

Grate cabbage, carrots and beets. Slice cucumber. Cut pepper
into rings. Slice or quarter tomatoes. Arrange cabbage, carrots
and beets in individual mounds or leaves. Surround by slices of
cucumber. Place rings of pepper and tomatoes on top. Place stalk
of celery on the side and serve. Serves two.

YOGURT DREAM SALAD

3 radishes, ½ cucumber, ½ green pepper,
2 scallions, 3 ozs. pot cheese, ½ cup yogurt
or clabbered milk.

Dice all vegetables, add pot cheese and yogurt. A few leaves of
watercress, cut up, goes well with this. If cucumber is scarce, substitute shredded green squash (zucchini). Serves one.

PEPPER SURPRISE

4 green or red peppers, ½ lb. cottage or pot
cheese, ½ cup seedless raisins, 2 large grated
apples.

Mix cheese, raisins and apples. Stuff peppers. Fine with relish
"Deluxe" or any other favorite relish or dressing. Serves four.

FRUIT SYMPHONY

2 tbs. raspberries, 2 tbs. blueberries, 3 tbs.
watermelon balls, 3 tbs. muskmelon balls, 1
ripe banana.

Place fruit on crisp lettuce leaves, place slices of banana around
it. Serve with pineapple juice as a dressing. Serves one.

RAISIN SPECIAL

1 small cabbage, 3 apples, 1 cup seedless
raisins. Lemon and oil dressing.

Soak raisins to soften them. Shred cabbage and apples into dressing to prevent discoloration. Add raisins and mix thoroughly.
Serve on lettuce leaves. Serves three.

WALDORF SALAD

1 cup shredded green cabbage, 1 cup
shredded green celery, 1 cup finely
shredded apple, ½ cup seedless raisins.

Mix and serve on green lettuce leaves. Serves two.

AN IDEAL SUMMER FRUIT LUNCH

1 cup blueberries, 1 cup raspberries, 1 cup bananas,
¼ cup papaya, 1 diced apple, 1 cup diced watermelon, ½ cup soaked raisins, 1 cup diced pears.

Place all in a deep bowl, pour over either pineapple juice or
diluted orange juice. Sprinkle a few sprigs of fresh parsley on top
for decoration. Serve with Ricotta or cottage cheese. Serves four.

FRUIT SALAD A LA KING

Diced banana, diced or cut up melon, diced apple, diced pear, diced avocado, a few raisins, with a dressing of pineapple juice. May be served with any soft bland cheese and makes an ideal lunch. Serves four.

Zestful Dressings, Relishes and Sauces

Many people enjoy eating their raw vegetables plain without any dressing. Once your taste buds begin to enjoy the fine flavors locked in the carefully chosen LIVE, RAW vegetables, no special dressings, seasonings or relishes are really required. But if you have not yet reached the point where you can enjoy raw vegetables in their natural state, I have no objection if the following healthful dressings, relishes or sauces are used to enhance the flavor of your salads:

AVOCADO DRESSING

Avocado, mashed, with the addition of lemon juice.
Avocado, mashed, with minced onions and lemon juice (to taste).

FRENCH DRESSING

¾ cup tomato juice, 1 or 2 tbs. soybean oil, juice of ⅓ lemon, half clove of garlic or a little grated onion. Shake well before serving.

SPECIAL FRENCH DRESSING

Soybean oil, lemon juice and honey—equal parts.

YOGURT DRESSING ROYALE

1 cup yogurt with 2 tbs. honey. Whip together. Makes a delicious dressing over raw-vegetable or fruit salad; stewed fruits and puddings.

BEET RELISH

Slice or dice cooked beets. Slice or dice raw onions. In a quart jar, add a layer of beets, then a layer of onions, until jar is filled. Add the juice of two lemons and a dash of raw sugar. Then fill jar with water and close tight. Let stand for several days.

RELISH DE LUXE

1 cup diced cucumber, ½ cup diced green ripe olives,
½ cup minced green pepper, ½ cup diced red radishes,
½ cup minced pimento, ¼ cup minced parsley.

Mix with tomato juice to which garlic and onion have been added.

ZEST DRESSING

½ cup soybean oil, 1 small grated onion, ½ tsp. honey
and ½ tsp. paprika.

Other Exciting, Easy-to-Make Dressings and Sauces

1. Mash ½ tomato (insides only) and ½ avocado and mix together.
2. Mash ½ banana with ½ avocado.
3. Mash ½ baked eggplant with a squirt of lemon juice.
4. 1 finely grated carrot and ½ squeezed lemon.
5. Mix one grated cucumber and ¼ avocado.
6. ½ cooked carrot and ½ cooked eggplant (mash together), add a few drops of lemon.
7. Juice 3 stalks of celery and mix with ¼ cut-up onion and 2 tablespoons of Ricotta cheese or cottage cheese.
8. Peel 2 apples and grate on a fine grater.
9. Mash ½ avocado and cut up ¼ onion in it.
10. Cut up ½ onion (diced), add 1 tablespoon soybean oil, juice of lemon.
11. Mash 1 cooked sweet potato, mash 1 cooked white potato, cut ¼ onion in and mix together.

Appetite's Delight: Steamed and Baked Vegetable Dishes

Always remember that the health- and blood-building raw vegetable salad comes first. You can eat it in combination with your baked potato, your natural brown rice, a small portion of any of the soft bland cheeses, or any other desirable protein food. Then if still hungry, any of the steamed or healthfully prepared vegetable dishes listed below can be added to round out the meal.

But make sure that you use them only if really hungry and make sure not to overeat!

MASTER RECIPE FOR VEGETABLE STEW

2 onions, 2 tomatoes or 1 cup of tomato juice.

Use tomato juice whenever possible, instead of water in cooking. Add a squirt of lemon juice and/or a sprinkling of vegetable broth powder if you desire it (available at health food stores). Add your favorite herbs if you like. This recipe can be used with the following vegetables: eggplant, zucchini (green Italian squash), young squash in yellow or white, string beans and peppers, beet tops and stalks, cabbage—both green and savoy, or any other vegetable you may desire to experiment with. The amount of onion and tomato can vary to taste.

A stew prepared as above can be eaten with either baked potatoes, sweet potatoes, carrots or parsnips or with baked pumpkin or hubbard squash.

A special delicacy can be had by cutting the acorn squash in halves, scooping out the seeds and filling with raisins and finely diced apples—bake for 20 to 25 minutes in a medium hot oven.

BAKED VEGETABLE DISH

1 bunch celery, 2 tomatoes or tomato juice,
¼ lb. green peas, ¼ lb. stringbeans, 1 small
eggplant, 1 carrot.

Dice celery, tomatoes, stringbeans, carrots. Wash eggplant. Dice with skin. Mix with peas and bake 25 minutes. Add oil just before serving. Serve with raw vegetable salad and brown rice or soybeans. Serves six.

CABBAGE SURPRISE

1 small green cabbage, 2 medium onions,
1 green pepper, 2 tomatoes (large), some
parsley or celery leaves.

Cut cabbage into 2 parts and steam until tender. Slice cabbage, onion, pepper, and tomatoes. Add minced parsley or celery leaves. Bake 20 minutes and serve with garlic and tomato juice dressing.

PIQUANT COMPANY LOAF

1 cup steamed green peas, 1 cup steamed
brown rice, 1 large Spanish onion, 3 carrots,
1 turnip, 1 parsnip, 1 knob celery (knob only),
¼ bunch parsley.

Steam rice for 20 minutes. Steam green peas separately for ten minutes. Steam carrots, turnips, parsley in a little water on a low flame until tender. Chop up onion and parsley and add to vegetables. Add peas and rice and mix. Bake in well oiled baking dish until browned. Serve with apple sauce or prunes. Serves six.

SPECIAL STUFFING

1 lb. green lima beans, 1 stalk celery, 1 grated
onion, 1 tbs. diced pimento, 1 tbs. soybean oil.

Steam lima beans, onions and pimento until almost tender. Mash all ingredients and use either to stuff green peppers, roll into cabbage leaves, roll as croquettes, or as a loaf. Bake ½ hour in medium oven. Serves two.

VEGETABLE DELIGHT

2 sweet potatoes, ½ lb. tart prunes, 1 bunch
small beets.

Scour prunes. Shred beets and potatoes. Pit prunes and cut into small pieces. Add the potatoes and beets. Steam for 25 minutes in 2 cups water. Serves four.

ASPARAGUS COMBINATION

½ lb. asparagus, ½ lb. green peas, 1 stalk celery,
½ cup tomato juice, 1 clove of garlic (grated).

Wash asparagus clean of all sand. Add green peas and celery with tomato juice and grated garlic. Steam or bake for 20 to 25 minutes. Serves two.

BAKED BEETS
6 medium beets.

Choose young tender beets. Scrub thoroughly with stiff vegetable brush. Bake until done (test with fork). Cut off ends and slice or dice. Serve on bed of crisp green lettuce leaves as salad with a dressing of fresh lemon or lime juice; or serve hot, peeled and sliced, adding a little oil and caraway seeds; or marinate in equal parts of water and lemon. Serves three.

HOT SWEET-SOUR BEETS
1 bunch cooked or baked beets sliced thin.

Marinate in juice of one lemon or one orange and one tablespoon of honey. Add thinly sliced onion. Keep in refrigerator for several hours before serving. Serves two.

STUFFED CABBAGE REVELATION
12 cabbage leaves (green—savoy cabbage preferred), 1 cup brown rice, ½ cup seedless raisins, 2 carrots, ½ cup green peas, 1½ cups tomato juice, 2 ripe tomatoes, 1 green pepper, 1 large onion, 2 cloves garlic, 2 tbs. honey.

Pour 6 cups of boiling water over brown rice and soak for 3–4 hours. Keep pot covered. Steam in same water over low flame until tender, then add honey. Soak cabbage leaves 15 minutes in boiling water to soften for rolling. Meanwhile chop fine or grind raisins, carrots and green peas together and mix with steamed rice.

Roll mixture in cabbage leaves, closing ends by folding the leaves inside. Cut up green pepper, slice onion, cut up tomatoes, grate garlic and add tomato juice. Steam 5 minutes. Drop in slowly the stuffed cabbage rolls, one at a time, into the mixture and continue to steam until tender, keeping pot covered. Serves six.

CORN CHOWDER

4 cobs of corn, 3 glasses of water, 4 carrots.

Cut kernels from cobs. Cut carrots into fine strips. Steam carrots 12 minutes. Add the corn. Steam 5 minutes more and serve. Serves four.

BAKED EGGPLANT WITH BROWN RICE

1 eggplant, 1 green pepper, 1 cup brown rice, 1 onion.

Cut raw eggplant into slices. Prepare rice by bringing to a boil in 6 cups of water and then let it stand with pot covered for half hour. Oil baking dish. Make layers of sliced onion, eggplant and green pepper. Sprinkle layers of brown rice on each layer of vegetables. Bake for about 30 minutes and serve with apple sauce or prunes. Serves four.

STEAMED KALE

1 lb. kale, 1 onion, 2 tomatoes.

Wash kale thoroughly to remove grit. Slice onion and tomatoes. Place in waterless cooker or steamer and steam until tender. Serves two.

OKRA STEW

1 lb. okra, 1 sweet potato, 1 stalk celery, 1 green pepper.

Slice potato and dice other vegetables. Stew until tender. Serve with brown rice (already cooked). Sprinkle vegetable broth powder when serving. Serves four.

STEAMED GREEN PEAS

1 lb. green peas in pods, 1 onion.

Steam peas in pods until almost done. Remove from pods and cook with sliced onion for 5 minutes longer. Sprinkle a little vegetable broth powder. Serve either hot or cold. Serves two.

POTATO-VEGETABLE PANCAKES

4 large potatoes, 2 carrots, 1 onion, ½ lb. squash, 2 tbs. vegetable oil, 2 tbs. vegetable broth powder.

Grate all ingredients on fine grater. Add vegetable broth powder and 1 tbs. vegetable oil. Pour into greased baking dish. Spread rest of oil over top and bake in hot oven for 15 minutes. Then lower flame and bake for 20 minutes more. Serves two.

POTATO PUDDING

6 potatoes, ½ cup chopped parsley, 4 large
scallions or 2 onions, 2 tbs. vegetable broth powder.

Pour boiling water on scrubbed potatoes, let stand for 5 minutes. Drain off water and peel off outer skin of potatoes and shred them. Chop scallions. Add parsley and vegetable broth powder. Bake in oiled pan until brown. Serves three.

POTATO LOAF

6 potatoes, 4 carrots.

Shred potatoes and carrots and mix. Sprinkle with vegetable broth powder. Bake in oiled pan 30 or 40 minutes, or until golden brown. Serve with apple sauce and an eggplant stew or a raw vegetable salad. Serves three.

SWEET POTATO LOAF

2 large sweet potatoes, 3 stalks of celery,
2 onions, 1 bunch parsley.

Scrub potatoes thoroughly. Bake for 15 minutes. Grate with the skin. Chop vegetables fine, add to grated potatoes and bake in slow oven in oiled dish for about ½ hour. Serve with relish, if desired. Serves four.

BAKED PUMPKIN

½ small pumpkin, 4 apples, 1 spoonful of honey.

Shred pumpkin and apples. Add honey and a sprinkle of cinnamon. Place in oiled baking dish. Bake 25 minutes. Serve with any stew desired or on a vegetable plate. Serves four.

BROWN RICE LOAF

1 cup brown rice, ½ bunch carrots, ¼ lb. stringbeans,
1 onion, ½ bunch celery.

Wash rice and soak overnight in enough water to cover. Boil for 20 minutes. Grind or grate onion, celery, stringbeans and carrots with skin after scrubbing them thoroughly. Mix with rice and bake for 30 minutes in oiled dish. Sprinkle paprika for color and flavor. Serve with favorite relish. Serves five.

STUFFED YELLOW SQUASH
(A favorite Florida Spa recipe)

Scrub squash with stiff brush. Cut off bottom ends and scoop out. Chop fine and add diced tomatoes, grated onion, finely minced green pepper and minced parsley. Add vegetable powder. Steam for a few minutes. Place in oiled baking pan and cover with a little oil. Then bake in medium oven until squash is tender. Serves one.

Nourishing Soups

The following soups may be used occasionally as a variation from the dishes regularly served.

A NOURISHING VEGETABLE SOUP

Steam 1 diced carrot, ½ cup peas, ½ cup broccoli, ½ cup celery, 1 potato, ½ eggplant, ½ onion, juice 2 stalks celery and carrots.

Mash steamed vegetables with potato masher, add fresh vegetable juice. Warm and serve. Serves four.

FLORIDA BEET SOUP

Cover 2 whole beets with water, boil until tender, then peel and grate, flavor gently with lemon juice. Used with boiled jacket potatoes, it makes a most desirable meal.

LENTIL SOUP

2 cups lentils (soaked), 3 carrots, 1 green pepper, ½ head celery.

Dice carrots, celery and pepper. Mix vegetables and lentils. Add 6 cups of water. Bring to a boil and simmer for 30 minutes. Serves six.

VEGETABLE BROTH

3 carrots, 1 green pepper, 1 onion, 1 potato,
1 small turnip, ½ knob celery, ½ cup parsley,
½ parsnip, 4 tbs. brown rice.

Clean and dice vegetables. Place into 6 cups of water. Bring to boil and simmer for 30 minutes. Steam or simmer rice separately for 20 minutes. Strain the vegetables and add the rice to the broth. Add vegetable broth powder or other seasonings. Serves six.

FRESH FRUIT SOUP

½ lb. cherries, 2 large peaches, 6 apricots,
6 plums, 2 tbs. honey, 4 glasses water.

Scald the peaches to remove skin. Remove from water and discard pits. Boil the 4 glasses of water and add fruits. Simmer for 25 minutes. Add honey and a little lemon juice to suit taste. Serves three.

GREEN PEA SOUP

1 cup green peas, 4 stalks green celery, 1 parsnip,
2 carrots, 1 large onion.

Dice all vegetables except peas, add 4 glasses of water, and bring to a boil. Put in green peas and simmer for 20 minutes. Add vegetable broth powder or any other flavoring desired. Serves four.

ONION SOUP

2 large onions, 1 large carrot, 1 green pepper,
½ cup brown rice (steamed).

Bring 6 cups of water to a boil. Dice carrot, pepper and onions. Mix with brown rice and put mixture into boiling water. Simmer for 30 minutes. Serves six.

POTATO SOUP

6 small potatoes, 1 onion, 2 stalks celery, 1 carrot.

Dice all vegetables. Add 3 cups of water. Bring to a boil and simmer for 30 minutes. Serve with a sprinkling of parsley greens and vegetable broth powder. Serves two.

Desserts and Puddings

A dessert to most people is something extra, something sweet or relishing with which to top off a full meal. But remember desserts are food, or should be food, and *good* food at that! And they should be eaten only if you are still hungry, not otherwise. And always bear in mind that the fewer the combinations at any one meal, the better.

CHERRY-APPLE DESSERT

1 lb. sweet cherries (or sour cherries with honey added after removing from stove), 2 lbs. apples.

Pit cherries. Peel, dice apples. Mix, steam 30 minutes. Sprinkle with nut meal if a richer dessert is desired. Serves four to six.

BAKED APPLES

4 apples, ½ cup seedless raisins.

Core apples, fill in with raisins in center. Place in baking dish and add glass of water. Bake for 25 minutes. Serve with honey or molasses, if additional sweetening is desired. Serves four.

GUEST STYLE BAKED APPLE

Take four apples and wash them thoroughly. Remove cores and peel one ring of skin off top. Fill in with blueberries or raisins and half teaspoonful of honey to each apple. Bake in a deep pan with ½ cup water. Baste apples occasionally with the juice in the pan. Medium oven for about 30 minutes. Sprinkle with coconut or chopped nuts. Serves four.

BANANA WHIP

Mash and whip two ripe bananas with fork. Add a few drops of lemon juice and ½ cup berries. Mix and serve.

RICE PUDDING

1 cup brown rice boiled, 2 tbs. honey,
½ cup soaked raisins, diced large apple. Mix
well, add another cup of water and bake in moderate
oven for 20 to 25 minutes.

A Résumé of Good Eating Habits

To help normalize your metabolism and restore internal cleanliness as a means of ridding your body of toxic wastes, keep remembering the following points:

1. Omit all sugars and all concentrated sweet foods. They are acid forming, rob the body of essential minerals and do much to impair bodily functioning.

2. Omit all iritating condiments and spices, as well as the highly stimulating and irritating foods and beverages. They are highly irritating to the digestive system, overexcite the nervous system, and place an added strain on the liver as well as on all the eliminative organs.

3. Limit your intake of dried fruits to just an occasional snack or treat. The naturally dehydrated apricots, peaches, nectarines, pears and prunes are best. All dried fruit should be sun-dried and not preserved or treated with sulfur dioxide or other chemicals. Sun-dried fruits are sold at most health food stores.

4. Omit fats of animal origin. This includes butter and cream. You may use vegetable oil, soybean oil, safflower oil, wheat germ oil, peanut oil—but even natural fats should be used sparingly. Select natural oils that are free from chemicals or preservatives. Avocados provide a choice form of fat, but never use any fat foods to excess. The avocado is an excellent source of vegetable or unsaturated fat.

5. Limit your intake of dairy foods to small amounts of Ricotta cheese, farmer cheese, pot cheese, cottage cheese or other soft bland cheeses. Be modest in your intake of clabber milk or yogurt. About four ounces of the soft bland cheese is usually sufficient for a meal.

6. Eliminate the use of all artificial bakery products and all foods that are made of bleached white flour and white sugar. Cakes, cookies, pastries, pies, macaroni, spaghetti, white breads and the like are to be shunned. These are health-destroying foods, and those who wish to rebuild and/or retain their health will do best to avoid them.

7. Baked potatoes, sweet potatoes, yams, corn on the cob, and natural brown rice are usually the carbohydrates to choose. They should be part of your daily meals. You may use millet, buckwheat groats and other whole grain foods, but remember that *moderation* is the watchword.

8. Since arthritis sufferers are usually deficient in vital minerals, the large raw vegetable salad, except when it cannot be handled by the body because of certain digestive or nervous disorders, is a *must*. Arthritis sufferers should enjoy large quantities of the green leafy vegetables, as well as the variety of the root vegetables. Carrots, beets, parsnips, turnips, kohlrabi and other root vegetables, sliced, cut into sticks, or finely grated for those who cannot eat them any other way, should make up the most essential part of the meal. Use a large raw vegetable salad at least once daily. Some have the idea that eating a raw vegetable salad daily could become tiresome, but after a while they begin to realize how nourishing and enjoyable it is. And with its many natural flavors because of the many varied vegetables that are used together, it can be a new sensation treat each time. To bring out the flavor of a raw vegetable salad, add lemon juice, a dressing of lemon juice and honey, or any of the wholesome, natural dressings I have listed above.

9. To promote a better assimilation of the foods you eat, omit desserts with the meal. Fresh or stewed fruits are desirable foods and may be used as a dessert if you are still hungry. Otherwise, omit them.

10. Watch your combinations! A large raw vegetable salad or a fresh fruit salad with a small portion of your favorite protein and one steamed vegetable, or a large raw vegetable salad with one of your favorite carbohydrate foods, plus one steamed vegetable, provides a *fine* meal. *The fewer the combinations eaten at*

any one time, the more thorough the assimilation and the more beneficial. Whatever you eat, let it be natural, wholesome foods. No other! And whenever possible use organically grown foods. Also, use foods in season, and again remember, use only those foods that help to rebuild the health and strength of your body.

EPILOGUE

We have now come to the end of this book. In a manner of speaking, it is really the beginning—a new life for the arthritis sufferer—a life that in time could free you entirely from your agonizing affliction. In this book, I have presented case after case of arthritis in its various forms and stages. I have shown you how the disease is most often traced to internal toxemia, accumulation of abrasive wastes, and the consequences of erroneous living. I have further explained how the arthritis sufferer can rid himself of this disease by internal cleansing and by joining in an alliance with the forces of Nature. It is the power of life within you that can uproot the disease and get you well. All you have to do is to provide the body with the care it needs, and the body slowly, gradually does the rest. The care you need to help you get well includes the use of natural health-building foods, regulated exercises, controlled fasting, the use of water therapy, cautious sunbathing, some manipulative help if obtainable, plus the various adjustments that you have to make in your way of living and thinking to bring about the required emotional control and a healthy outlook on life. All of these are natural and drugless means of restoring health. I have employed these measures during a lifelong practice working with countless thousands of arthritis cases with excellent results. These measures marshaling the healing powers of your own body help to restore body balance, bring about a restoration of normal metabolic functioning, and in this way help to reestablish normal health. Arthritis can be uprooted and cast out of the system, but it can be done only when you work with the forces of your own body—with the forces of nature, not against them.

Now as I look back to more than a half century of practice,

thinking of the countless thousands of so-called "hopeless" arthritis cases who by adopting this plan of care and adhering to it faithfully have succeeded in regaining their health, I can well understand why so many keep singing the praises of this method and keep urging others to turn to it for the help they need. "With your guidance, I have found my way back to health. You showed me how to do it, you encouraged me to keep up with this care, and now I am well again. Life is wonderful. Life once more is worth living." How often have I heard this or something similar said to me. Results have not always come easily, but what a joy when I keep thinking of the innumerable thousands who have come to me crippled and full of despair and who by adhering to this program have discovered that arthritis is not an incurable disease, that with good care arthritis sufferers can get well!

The techniques and measures that I have employed throughout my many years of practice with such phenomenal success have been presented in this book. Just as they have helped many thousands of others, so they can help you. Give yourself the chance you need—work with Nature. Join the many thousands who have found freedom from arthritis by resorting to these drugless, natural means. Adopt my plan, adhere to it, and a glorious and healthy new life will be your reward. Be happy, be healthy and —stay well!

INDEX

215

"Keep in touch, would you, this time?"

Longarm grinned at him. It was one of Billy's pet peeves. No matter how often one of Vail's deputies telegraphed progress reports, the man was never satisfied. Longarm often had the sneaking suspicion that Billy still thought of himself as a field man and was probably convinced that he could have done a better job if he'd been out there himself.

"I always do," Longarm said happily, and escaped through the office door before Billy Vail could offer a retort to that perfectly obvious untruth. There were times, in fact, when Deputy Marshal Custis Long took a positive delight in twitting his boss by remaining silent during the course of an investigation. Not that he would withhold information. He would not think of doing something that might jeopardize the job he was assigned to do, and a man never knew when unexpected circumstances—like knives, clubs, or bullets—might make it necessary for another deputy to step into the middle of a job only partially done. But damned if Longarm was going to go out of his way just to say howdy three times a day, the way Billy would have liked them all to do.

Longarm paused at the top of the federal building steps to light a cheroot, then hurried down into Colfax Avenue in search of a hack.